In the Lyme-Light

Portraits of Illness and Healing

For the malicont. Wort Family

from Sarah + Dick

Emily Bracale

Emily used to be a teacher at Isleford. years ago.

Emily Bracale

To all those who have helped me,
to all those still in need of help,
may blessings of healing
and happiness
come to all.

Self Published by Emily Bracale
Maine Authors Publishing and Cooperative
558 Main Street
Rockland, ME 04841

Copyright 2011 by Emily Bracale
Foreword copyright 2011 by Patricia L. Gerbarg, MD

ISBN: 978-1-936447-99-2

Foreword

My first reactions to *In the Lyme-Light* were surprise, recognition, and gratitude. I was surprised by the eloquence of Emily's visual images and the beauty in her description of the devastating effects of Lyme disease on her mind, body, and spirit. Those of us who have lived with Lyme disease, who have struggled to understand and express what we experience, recognize exactly what Emily portrays in words and colors. And with that recognition comes a sense of gratitude that someone has found a way to tell our story, to convey the many nuances of denying, resisting, hiding, self-doubting, trying, loving, learning, adapting, and eventually coping with a mysterious and widely misunderstood illness.

As a physician, my concerns about Lyme disease began as I saw the number of deer increase every year in our neighborhood. Like many families, we had a little dog, Rocky. Like many pets Rocky wore a pest repellent collar and still brought deer ticks into our house. Being a conscientious mother, I meticulously removed Rocky's ticks and scoured the house for any that might have fallen off, never thinking that I might be the one to get bitten.

As with Emily, Lyme took its time creeping into my system causing a little soreness here, a little stiffness there and gradually over about five years, more and more pain, weakness, exhaustion, and mental clouding. Emily's painting, "Rock Bottom," says it all. When you are curled up in bed for hours waiting for the pain to stop, unable to think clearly, fighting off fears that you might never get your life back, fending off doubts that this could all be in your head, feeling guilty about being sick…you are just a rock at the bottom of an endless dark sea.

Although Lyme devastated my life during the last two years of my illness, I consider myself lucky because an infectious disease specialist finally diagnosed the condition based on a SPECT scan of my brain, that is a special scan that showed where the narrowing of blood vessels (from Lyme organisms invading the inner lining) was reducing blood flow to critical brain areas. After nine months of antibiotic treatment I began what is now about 15 years of post-Lyme gradual recovery. Although the antibiotics were necessary to eradicate the infection, they did not repair the damage it had done to the cells of my brain, muscles and tendons. Antibiotics did not stop the inflammatory process that is much quieter now, but that still smolders in my tendons and that is too easily evoked by any strenuous activity. Fortunately, my husband, Dr. Richard Brown, had developed considerable expertise in complementary treatments. One of the herbs he tried, *Rhodiola rosea*, restored my balance, memory, and other cognitive functions. Some of the medicinal compounds in the roots of this herb enhance cellular energy production and repair. Discovering the benefits of this herb was the genesis of my interest in complementary and alternative medicine. This led to an entirely new direction in my career and the many rewards of being able to heal people who could not respond to other treatments. With *Rhodiola rosea*, other supplements, and mind-body practices, I am still not able to do everything I used to do, but I can do anything that is really important for me, my family, and my work.

One of my favorite pictures is Emily's "Pillows." It reminded me of the nine pillows I used to need in order to sleep during the worst of times. It made me laugh and feel good about the fact that now I only need two.

When Lyme infection is recognized quickly, a three-week course of antibiotics is usually all that is needed. However, only about 40% of people bitten by ticks develop the tell-tale bull's-eye rash and only about 70% show positive results on standard blood tests for Lyme. That leaves thousands who may not know they were bitten or whose cases were untreated due to false negative tests. Many of these people are at risk for developing long term complications including chronic pain, inflammation, fatigue, insomnia, cognitive slowing, memory loss, incoordination, loss of balance, brain damage, heart damage, paralyses of nerves, digestive problems, rashes, and more. Lyme disease is the Great Pretender. Since the microorganisms can invade any tissues anywhere in the body, the damage they cause can mimic many other illnesses. When a patient has odd symptoms that don't fit into a standard pattern, doctors may assume that the problem is psychological.

Now that I have become a "Lyme literate" psychiatrist, many Lyme patients are sent to me because their medical doctors believe that their symptoms are psychosomatic, that is "all in the patient's head." Well, some of the symptoms may be in the patient's head because that is one of the favorite locations for Lyme spirochetes. For example, an infectious disease doctor treated a college student with Lyme disease for one month with antibiotics. After stopping the antibiotics, the doctor sent this student to see me because he was having mood swings and acting strangely. A brain scan showed a long, thin cavity in the brain tissue in the right cerebral hemisphere. The other doctor thought it might have been caused by an unknown brain injury. However, there was no history of brain injury and the cavity was nowhere near any of the brain areas that are damaged during most kinds of head trauma. By reminding my colleague that infections in brain cavities are highly resistant to antibiotics, I was able to persuade him to resume and maintain the antibiotics. Within a week, the patient began to recover.

Two of the most essential ingredients for Lyme recovery are to develop a fighting spirit and a way to transform the experience, to make it part of your pattern of personal growth so that it enriches your life. As with anything that is an unwanted part of us, the more we avoid, deny, reject, and hate it, the more it drains our spirit. Seeing Lyme for what it is, accepting that it is an integral part of our existence, and using all of our awareness, insight, and creative energy to learn from it and to ultimately transform the experience and ourselves is the deeper message within this book. This is the "Letting Go," the letting go of one's natural fearful, defensive reaction to pain and suffering in order to explore the possibilities of creating an existence you never envisioned for yourself. By sharing her story, Emily the teacher leads us to the question, "Can we find a way through our disease to live a better life and nurture the spirit of love within ourselves and those who are dear to us?"

I hope that readers will share this book with as many people as possible, not only to heighten awareness and understanding for those who live with Lyme, but also because prevention is one of the best weapons we have in fighting what is currently a losing battle against the growing epidemic of Lyme. For example, in places where vigorous public education about Lyme prevention was implemented the number of new Lyme cases dropped by as much as 70%.

Medical debates, battles over insurance coverage for antibiotics, absence of serious public health initiatives, attacks on doctors who recognize and treat chronic Lyme, and lack of accurate tests and effective treatments all contribute to the private and public burden of this disease. Many Lyme patients are left with no doctor, no insurance coverage, and no treatment as their illness relentlessly progresses. Sometimes families who cannot understand the illness or who cannot bear to be around the person who is ill, abandon their loved one, leaving them without financial, physical, or emotional support. I believe that this book will contribute to the growing literature on Lyme disease, not only as an artistic statement, but also as a medium that may open peoples' eyes and hearts to the inner world of those who are experiencing a life-changing illness.

My hope is that as more people come to understand the impact of Lyme on all of our lives, the tide will turn in the direction of more enlightened education, treatment, and prevention. I just want to thank Emily for sharing her extraordinary book with me.

Patricia L. Gerbarg, MD
Assistant Professor of Clinical Psychiatry
New York Medical College
Co-author of "How to Use Herbs, Nutrients and Yoga in Mental Health Care" (W.W. Norton, 2009)
www.haveahealthymind.com

Introduction

Someday this book may become obsolete. Sooner rather than later I hope. For now, I regret to say, it still has a role to play. Although this story is about one person, it illustrates the experiences of thousands of others: the experience of Lyme disease. It shares the impact of Lyme on my inner and outer life and the process of healing that began to lift me out of that nightmare and into a new life. I'm sharing it for the sake of those who may be able to avoid this particular nightmare altogether by becoming more aware. This book is also for those who are ill, "in the Lyme-Light" as it were, and for their supporting cast – partners, relatives, parents, teachers, doctors, friends, counselors, co-workers – anyone whose life and relationships may be tinted by the effects of Lyme. This book may help you communicate your experience to other people, or it may help you witness the Lyme experience from an insider's perspective. It may offer some new ideas. For some people it may serve as a wake up call, for others as an uncomfortable challenge to denial.

As some of you already know firsthand, there is much controversy in the realm of Lyme disease – medically, scientifically, politically, and legally. Other people are bringing those aspects to the public's awareness. My wish is to participate as an artist, from my heart, sharing with you a self-portrait of my particular experience. Having been an artist, writer, and teacher for most of my life, it was natural for me to turn to paints, words, and stories to come to terms with my experience of illness. And this expression, in turn, has been an integral part of my personal healing process. Now the result goes out as this book to serve whatever purpose it may for the sake of other people.

Here is how it began: By early 2009, my life consisted of treading water from minute to minute, hour to hour – getting through breakfast, getting to lunch, getting to dinnertime, getting the kids to bed, finally lying down but not sleeping well; too much anxiety, weird electrical buzzing sensations, crazy unfocused thoughts, and chronic physical pain. I frequently felt so miserable that I wanted to leave my body. Yet no one realized how sick I had become because gradually, over seven years, I had dropped out and drifted away from almost all intimate contact with other people. For many years (for many reasons) I largely avoided seeking medical help (other than for the birth of my second child in 2003). I knew something was terribly wrong but I certainly didn't suspect that Lyme disease was a part of it.

Until that year, I knew very little about the disease – I assumed things, heard of people getting it, but never bothered to ask them what that meant. They, being down with it, didn't have much energy to volunteer. So I hadn't yet identified my symptoms with a disease, nor even admitted to myself that I was so physically ill.

Many people who think they have Lyme have had a difficult time getting support and treatment. Some are told that they are imagining part or all of the predicament. Some are resigned to treating Lyme as an unfortunate lifelong affliction that they must just cope with. Some are told they have a mental illness or emotional issues in need of counseling and therapy. What stands out about my story is that I was the one who tried to make the disease be "all in my head" for so many years, treating my symptoms as psychosomatic side effects of stress and "personal issues." I ignored the escalating severity of physical and neurological problems until there was considerable damage to the nervous system and a compromised immune system. By early 2009 my physical, social, personal, financial, and professional life had all "bottomed out." Even my lifelong love of making art was gone. It felt as if my old life was over, but I couldn't see any future.

Then that April, through a series of fortunate events, I began to suspect that I might have Lyme disease – and possibly had for half my life! I began a crash course in learning about the disease and how to self-advocate for the treatment I needed. I was astonished to learn how serious Lyme could become and that it is a subject of incredible controversy. I began trying to share what I was going through with family, friends, and doctors, cautiously revealing some of the darker side of my life for the first time. Talking with other Lyme patients let me know that I was going down the right path. After asking about my symptoms one called me a "poster child" for Lyme and told me to seek medical help immediately. Finding out about Lyme disease was frightening, but it was also an epiphany, a light in the darkness, a sudden "lightening of the karmic load." It explained so much. I felt as if I were waking up from a long and crazy nightmare.

Starting treatment that summer made enormous positive changes but it didn't exactly make my body feel "all better" right away, since so much was out of balance. However, I knew I was in recovery when ideas for this art and writing began coming to mind. One evening after a long hot bath I jotted down a whole page of notes describing how to illustrate symptoms symbolically. Using acrylic paints on birch plywood I started painting. As physical healing commenced, this creative project turned my attention toward affirming life.

But there was still fatigue, contending with medications and their side effects, two part-time jobs, and endless household tasks as a single parent of a preschooler and a teenager. At some point, feeling too flat, gray, and overwhelmed "to ever be creative again," I threw the list away.

Then, in January of 2010, the urge to paint came back in force – almost compelling me to attend, no matter how tired and achy I still felt. When I let go of trying to figure out how to do anything and just showed up, so did the inspiration. The art that emerged was different from any I'd done before. Most of my work had been careful representations of outdoor scenes, and cultural scenes from traveling. The new work portrayed internal landscapes and internal journeys. Many images held meaning beyond what I was aware of to begin with, and humor beyond what I felt consciously capable of inventing. Sometimes I found myself laughing out loud as if it were someone else's ideas I was discovering, tapping into that delightful zone of being the radio, broadcasting songs, instead of trying to be the station, figuring out what to play. As I experienced the creation of each piece and studied each board, it became clear that I needed to add some written explanations, so I started writing as well. This was a hugely satisfying process of expression and discovery.

I also sensed that my story was meant to be shared – that it could play some role in awakening awareness. Any time I questioned the wisdom of revealing so much detail from my private (and often uncomfortable) experiences, I sensed an inner "green light" to continue. Just two months later, at the end of February 2010, twenty-six paintings and eighteen pages of notes became the first Lyme-Light exhibit, held at College of the Atlantic in Bar Harbor, Maine. It was a big "coming out" experience. Much of what I shared was news to my family, friends, and neighbors. People in the community had known me as a student at the college, an elementary school teacher, a private art teacher, a home schooling parent, and an artist who painted watercolor landscapes. Now I shared publicly what I had recently been afraid to admit even to myself.

Paradoxically, the degree to which the work was subjective and personal was the degree to which it made an impact. Word spread and people asked for interviews, a website, a book. Many people with Lyme or who had friends and family with Lyme said that this story resonated with their own experiences. The bizarre descriptions and images I shared met with grateful exclamations of recognition. Several people decided to get tested or seek treatment. A friend offered to create a website for the work. Sharing my story made me let go of a tight hold on individual suffering and put me in touch with a sense of

connectedness and strength. Many people have shared their own stories and encouragement in return. I feel that we're pioneers in the larger story of Lyme, giving "Lyme-Light" new meaning. We're bringing to light our own stories, and offering the light of awareness to our communities far and wide. Sometimes, if only briefly, we're able to model a hopeful, faithful, and light-hearted acceptance of our condition as we work to improve it, having discovered (by traveling such a difficult path) that we needed to let go of some of our old beliefs and habits that were further weighing us down. A potential positive side effect of Lyme disease for everyone is that it challenges us to develop more honesty, persistence, and courage, as well as humor, patience, and cooperation. Without these, the suffering can be unbearable. With these, there may be healing on many levels.

While this book focuses on Lyme disease, it also touches on dynamics of illness and healing that could apply to other illnesses. I believe that all illnesses take place on many levels simultaneously. Lyme is just a part of a much larger story. But through facing Lyme specifically, I have touched down into all the areas of my life that have been neglected and in need of healing; physically, emotionally, mentally, socially, and spiritually. This has been, and continues to be, an immensely powerful process of transformation on all levels. By now I have learned and grown and benefitted from the process so deeply that it is impossible to see myself as a victim any more.

Yet I feel the deepest sympathy and compassion for those who are still down in the mire of symptoms, too enmeshed to imagine a way through. Insanity sucks. Pain sucks. I know this. But you are not alone, and there may be new support which you can yet find.

I offer this book in the spirit of encouragement. I wish to encourage people to do their own research and take care of themselves and each other as best they can. I wish to encourage sincere listening and honest communication about Lyme disease and our personal struggles with it. Perhaps this book will encourage some people to erase lines they may have drawn in the sand and perhaps open to a new perspective they find healing – physically, emotionally, mentally, socially, and spiritually.

The most hopeful thing I have to say at this time is that now, when I read about the worst of it, my story seems to be about a different person. I have a new life; I've come that far.

Best wishes to all

Emily Bracale
Bar Harbor, Maine
January 11, 2011

1. Lime-aid

"If life gives you limes, make limeade." This illustration is a metaphor for many things: it refers to the therapeutic act of transforming my difficult experiences of Lyme disease into art and words that communicate to other people. Perhaps this project will aid others. The contents of the bag could also represent donations of time, money, and support from friends and family helping me with personal expenses and supporting this Lyme-Light project.

Some people call it "Lymes," but it's officially "Lyme" disease. That name comes from the place, Lyme, Connecticut, where a woman like me started asking questions, telling her stories, and believing that more attention and support was needed for the strange illness suddenly afflicting so many people in her community. The term "Lyme disease" can refer to one family of bacteria, *Borrelia burgdorferi (Bb)*, which has many different strains and is a cousin of syphilis. (In some reports it is called "deer syphilis.") It can be passed to humans and other mammals through the bite of certain ticks and is also known to be spread by migrating birds such as Canada Geese. Pets can also bring ticks into the home. Some studies discuss other methods of *Bb* transmission via mosquitos and fleas, and by gestational and sexual transmission from person to person. By now cases of Lyme have been reported in all states and in many countries around the world. Some reports consider *Bb* infection to be a global epidemic.

The term "Lyme disease" is also (inaccurately) used more broadly to refer to the varied cocktail of other tick-borne diseases (TBD's) a person may acquire from a bite, such as Ehrlichiosis and Babesiosis, a protozoan disease similar to malaria. These may also be referred to as "co-infections." Furthermore, it is hypothesized that an immune system compromised by *Bb* and other TBD's may be vulnerable to other infections, such as yeast infections and chronic herpes outbreaks, which have nothing to do with ticks or *Bb*, and these may also be referred to as "co-infections." One chronic illness might upset hormonal balances, which in turn might lead to other illnesses. In an immune-compromised body, a "passing" cold or yeast infection might take root and last for months. The

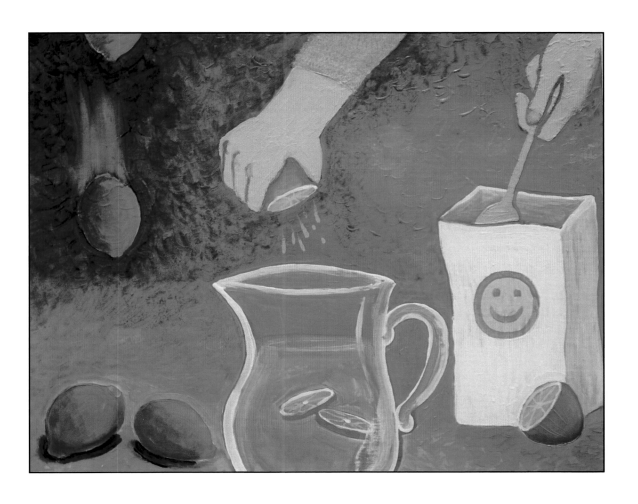

1. Lime-aid
acrylic on birch
16" x 20", 2010

situation can become a complicated mess both symptomatically and verbally!

The good news is that not all ticks are carriers, not everyone bitten becomes ill, and some who do may heal on their own; it is not necessarily going to develop into a chronic disease. But it is good to become more educated about the signs and symptoms. Two of the greatest risk factors in getting a chronic, costly, and debilitating case of Lyme disease are denial – of its existence and potential severity – and lack of awareness and prevention. The sooner the disease is suspected, diagnosed, and treated, the better and cheaper the outcome is for everyone. But we're still in the pioneering phase. The common blood tests are not always accurate. A person may be very ill and have Lyme but get a negative blood test for many reasons. Until recently, I, like many people, did not realize that Lyme disease could be so serious. Aware or not, anyone who plays outside in nature, gardens, hikes, or sits out in grassy fields painting as I often used to do, is a potential candidate for Lyme.

For more information I recommend the website for ILADS: the International Lyme and Associated Diseases Society, at www.ilads.org.

2. "Fine, thanks!"

In March, 2009, when I turned forty-two, I made my first appointment in six years for a routine physical. "How are you?" my new doctor asked. "Fine," I replied politely, same as to most people in passing. I did mention having trouble sleeping, feeling worn down, roving aches and pains, becoming easily agitated and irritable. But I said all this kind of "off to the side," muffled by self-conscious embarrassment. After all, what single mother of two home schooled kids (preschool and teen) after five months of a Maine winter isn't a bit frazzled? I was wary of coming across as a complainer. At a rare outing with other moms and kids I casually mentioned just wanting to "walk away from it all." That was one of my rare "squeaks," referring delicately to suicide. "Don't we all?" someone replied. I didn't say anything more.

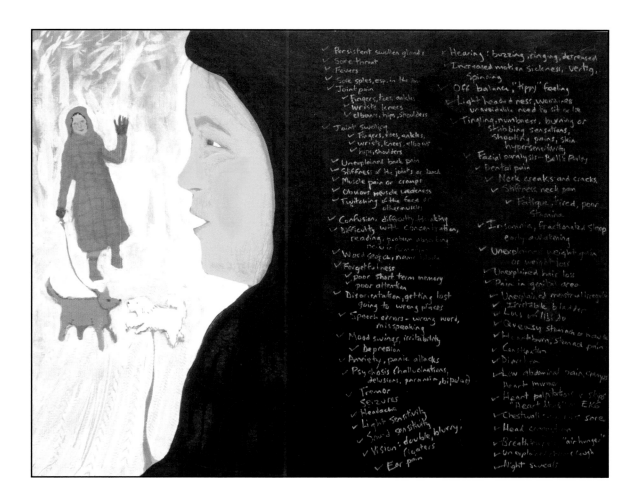

2. "Fine, thanks!"
acrylic and chalk pencil on birch
16" x 20", 2010

There is a silencing process inherent in having an undiagnosed chronic illness. If you have an acute case of flu you stay in bed, don't brush your hair, let the raggedness show. Anyone could tell that you are ill. But when the feeling of being ill goes on for weeks, months, years – waxing and waning in erratic cyclical patterns – you learn to somehow carry on to the best of your ability. You get dressed up for work, brush your hair, put on a social smile. There are bills to pay, children to raise, friends and neighbors with more acute surgeries and chemotherapy appointments to attend to. If at times you acknowledge the depth of the physical pain you are enduring, your mind gone madly blank or streaming with hallucinations, the fact that you feel like crying all the time and sometimes do (when there is a private moment – it's like peeing; you can wait, but it's gotta come out sometime) – you can start to question your own sanity around it. Are you, in fact, going crazy? A hypochondriac? A lazy person looking for excuses? Or, worst of all, are you committing some kind of New Age Error by manifesting all this instead of good health?

My symptoms confused me. Sometimes I was fine for a few weeks. I often thought it was because I was doing something right: eating the right food, getting enough sun and exercise, thinking positive thoughts. Then, for no apparent reason, I'd get wrung out again: mentally, emotionally, and physically. I suspected arthritis, chronic fatigue, and fibromyalgia, but friends and family with those conditions didn't seem to get relief from going to their doctors, so I didn't even bother asking. Once, three years after my son was born, I went for one pelvic exam since I was feeling the most excruciating pain in my life – as if a barbed knitting needle were up my spine – and was told I had a vaginal yeast infection. Soon, as usual, blisters broke out in my private parts, but I did not test positive for herpes. The visit and tests cost me a month's income. This episode remained part of the mystery which I found too frustrating and far too expensive to research further. I didn't have health insurance since I'd resigned from my job as a teacher, and I wasn't earning much money being at home with my children, so I tried to make the best of it all on my own.

I also feared being a drag on friends and family by admitting how miserable I often felt. Cultural conditioning upheld my silence. "If you don't have something nice to say, don't say anything at all." "Keep a stiff upper lip." "Be self sufficient." "Keep trying harder." I tried so hard to be demure that it's no wonder people took it lightly. Their response became an element in the vicious cycle of denial: as other people's minimization became internalized, I "normalized" my symptoms even as they became more serious. I felt ashamed about complaining, thinking other people must be enduring the same conditions (but so much better than I) and that I was weak for making such suffering out of "normal" life. After all, everybody gets sore sometimes, many parents are sleep-deprived, and many people seem "stressed out" these days.

What got me to "peep" louder was starting to learn how serious Lyme disease could become – not just some minor arthritis in the knees as I had once thought. Lyme is capable of producing a broad range of symptoms in different parts of the body. I read that, if left untreated, it could lead to brain lesions, organ failure, paralysis, dementia, and death. Some people who had been diagnosed as having severe anemia, leukemia, chronic fatigue syndrome, fibromyalgia, rheumatoid arthritis, lupus, multiple sclerosis, Parkinson's, and ALS experienced significant improvement when their condition was found to include or even be caused by Lyme disease and other tick borne diseases, and therefore was treatable through antibiotics. I also learned that symptoms of Lyme could wax and wane. I began to see how the seemingly unrelated symptoms I had endured on and off for many years could all be part of one larger picture.

The words on the dark side of this painting are from the paper "Advanced Topics In Lyme Disease: Diagnostic Hints And Treatment Guidelines For Lyme And Other Tick Borne Illnesses," by Joseph J. Burrascano Jr., M.D. (2008). As I began to suspect that I had Lyme, I began talking with other people in my community who had it. They asked about my symptoms and then told me I was a "poster child" for it and to seek treatment immediately. The urge to cry out for help finally trumped my stoic silence and old fashioned "good manners."

3. Depression

Depression can be an illness onto itself, but it can also be a side effect of a physical illness. I fell into it several time a year for many years, but it always seemed to be in reaction to some condition beyond my control. Although tending to be a quiet, serious, and studious person, I didn't think of myself as a pessimistic or "depressed person" per se. During the good periods, I was perfectly capable of finding beauty and meaning in life. The pattern was that for a while I would feel creative, inspired, invested in my career, in love with my family, and perceive myself to be a well-adjusted, intelligent, and highly functioning adult with a positive outlook on life. Then, unexpectedly, the bottom would drop out. I'd begin to feel lethargic, fatigued, unmotivated, sore, achy, arthritic, anxious, angry, spaced out, and stupid – not able to organize thoughts well or feel a sense of capability for carrying out the kinds of complex creative projects that made my life interesting. Inspiration and confidence would disintegrate, and I'd feel as if I'd fallen into a deep hole with no way out, or flipped over in a kayak that I couldn't right. There was only waiting – for weeks usually – before the sky would appear again. Then there was grief over lost time, a toll on my projects and relationships, and frustration about seeming to have so little control.

From 2001 to 2009 there was more falling and less rising as the cycles continued. The randomly occurring debilitating symptoms and lack of a sense of moving forward with my life on any front led to despondency and desperation. Twice during that period I sought medication for depression, but both times the person I consulted helped me conclude that I was a strong courageous woman with challenging life circumstances, but not clinically depressed.

This painting evolved from an idea to paint the form of a person in blue with an amorphous blue background. The first figure I rendered looked too cartoonish to symbolize depression, so I took a big brush and began swirling the wet paint into the background. Quickly a new figure emerged, a phantom from within the paint itself. I did a bit of work bringing it into completion, but the larger part of the composition lay in recognizing what had spontaneously emerged beyond my

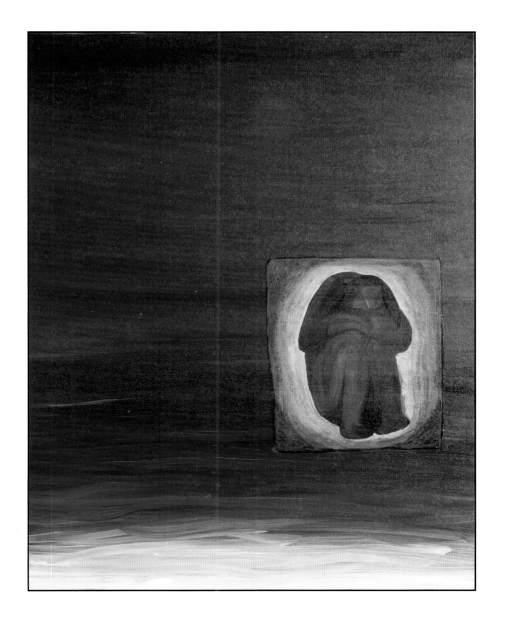

3. Depression
acrylic on art board
16" x 20", 2009

conscious efforts – and letting it be. Herein lies a lesson from the experience of being ill; it's simply a fact that I can't control as much as I thought I could, and what I can control is on the inside more than the outside. Much of "what works out" does so because I've opened up to seeing it in a different way, not because I've understood how to make it work better through my willful efforts. A positive side effect of being so ill for so long is that it caused me to consider new ways of viewing myself. Who is the "me" who thinks she has to have control? What observes, unperturbed, even as "I" appear to be suffering? In spite of physical setbacks there can still be soulful progress. The figure in the painting seems to be alone and suffering, yet she is surrounded by light and floating.

4. Rock Bottom

Rock Bottom was the first image that came to mind to paint, giving form to the formless experience of fatigue and having "bottomed out" in so many ways. For years I looked outward and blamed life circumstances for inducing symptoms of stress and fatigue – divorce, returning to full time work, remarriage, pregnancy, separation, unmedicated birth of a 10 lb. 14 oz. baby, nursing around the clock, a second divorce, home schooling two highly creative children, moving four times in six years, job loss, financial strain.

I also blamed myself, thinking if only I could learn to deal with stress better and have a more positive attitude, then I'd feel better. Gradually, in spite of my best efforts, things just kept falling apart – not only my career, intimate relationships, and family connectedness, but also my inner life. What I clung to as foundational beliefs kept failing to make life feel better. Whenever I adopted a new spiritual or philosophical mind set to help me interpret what was going on and navigate through it, it might have some useful effect for a little while, but ultimately could not hold me together through the next phase of debilitating symptoms. The bottom just kept falling out.

While it is true that life circumstances were a source of stress, the other hidden side of the circle was that a physical disease was strongly influencing every aspect of my life. I noticed friends and neighbors encountering births, deaths, job

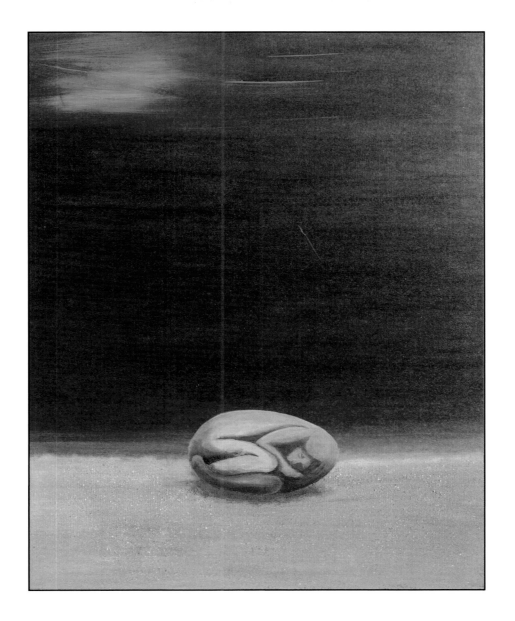

4. Rock Bottom
acrylic and sand on art board
16" x 20", 2009

changes, and divorces – going through stressful periods – but having the physical stamina and internal coherence to manage these changes and go on with their lives in a vibrant way. In comparison, I felt like a person riding a bicycle on the shoulder of the freeway. Eventually I became so ill that there was no capacity left for "trying harder" to "make things work" anymore. That was the turning point.

Although the idea of falling can have negative connotations – giving up, failure, loss of control, disgrace – it can also be about surrender, letting go of resistance. The experience of bottoming out can be full of grace and positive potential. There is relief in having landed. One has finished for now. Dying? Waiting? Who knows what is to come? There is rest, at last. Perhaps that is the only choice any more, so it is finally allowed to happen. There is relief in total surrender.

Perhaps the figure in the rock/egg is gestating, going through metamorphosis. To signify that the scene was under water I sprinkled sand onto the wet paint and added a few strokes of green to the upper left as if light were shining through it.

Adding a touch of this green to the top of the figure revealed the idea to me (I didn't know it going in) that, although she appeared to be alone, there was a healing presence – green light or energy – reaching her through the dark water. Thus was the title for the exhibit conceived.

5. One Step at a Time

In late April 2009, after visiting relatives in the Berkshires, I noticed a little pink dot above my ankle which expanded into a two inch wide red circle with a bruised, blistery center. It didn't hurt, but itched enough to make me notice. That was the first clue. It looked like a bull's eye to me. I went back to my doctor. She didn't think it was a Lyme rash because of the bruise and the fact that it itched, but she sent out a blood test to see.

Next clue: at the library I noticed a new book on the table called *Cure Unknown, Inside the Lyme Epidemic* by Pamela Weintraub (2009). I hadn't gone to the library consciously seeking information about Lyme disease (believing I already

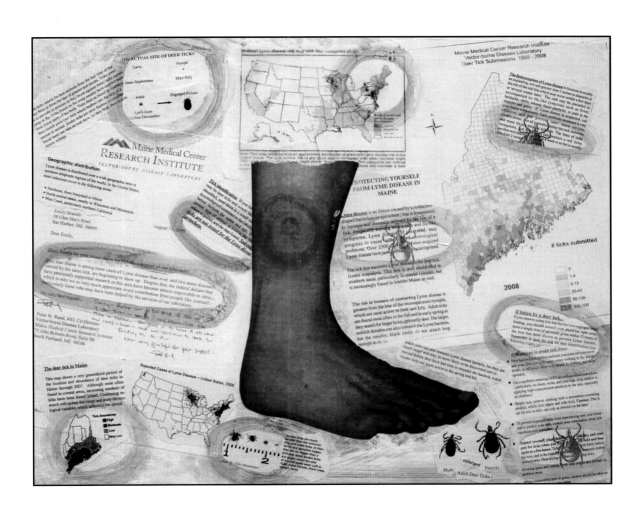

5. One Step at a Time
acrylic and paper collage on birch
16" x 20", 2010

knew what it was and wasn't), nor had I had the focus or stamina to read adult nonfiction books for a long time, but I felt drawn to check the book out. Pouring through it over the next 36 hours was a revelatory experience. The more I read, the more I made the connection between the stories of people with chronic Lyme disease and my own symptoms going back for many years.

Although (as it turns out) I have always lived in potentially tick-infested areas and have spent much time lingering in nature, such as when painting scenic views, I never knew to check for ticks. I also had no idea how large (or small) they could be. Memories began to resurface of times I thought I had a splinter – when I had picked and poked at a tiny black dot, trying in vane to squeeze it out. From having gardened, I made the association between that kind of splinter which is embedded straight in and looks like a pinpoint, and times when I'd gotten a rose briar or thorn stuck in my leg. Now I believe those "splinters" were really embedded ticks. Instead of a one shot deal, I saw myself as having had multiple exposures over many years. I also learned there could be no rash at all, or other (non-bull's eye) rashes from the other tick borne diseases, even years later.

Over the next month I became sicker and sicker, but in all the same ways that I had felt on and off for years. It was frightening enough to keep my attention focused and help me do things out of character such as pestering the front desk at the clinic with one message after another, asking if the test was back (it was negative), asking for another test (also negative), explaining in a letter that this was typical for long term cases, writing and hand delivering an eight page letter about my symptoms, getting a referral to another doctor, and asking to start antibiotics while waiting for that first appointment. I felt my health declining back into the craziest of prior low points. My spine felt electric and "buzzy" inside. There was so much swelling in my joints and tail bone area that it limited my natural stride. Walking two blocks to the library and back left me flat and exhausted for the rest of the day. I had a relentless pressure headache, dizziness, tipsiness like being slightly drunk, trouble judging distances, and I frequently tripped on the stairs in my small house. I narrowly avoided three car accidents from overlooking the approach of other cars while trying to drive across streets in my small town neighborhood. My bones and muscles ached like an acute case of the flu. Holding a telephone up to my ear for a three minute conversation felt like holding a difficult yoga pose that burned. I was short of breath and felt like crying all the time.

The appointment with the Lyme Aware doctor kept getting moved back for various necessary reasons until the first week in July. During May and June, the round rash slowly receded until all that was left was a bruise. (One year later it was still visible and tender.) During those two months I began to wake up from my own denial and to assemble facts and figures to get other people's attention. It was exasperating and empowering. It got me to stand up for myself more than I ever had before.

6. Fluff and Icebergs

Coming out of denial and into acknowledgement of my body's condition was a back and forth process. Before I got the validation of a doctor's diagnosis, I wavered between worrying I was making up a story – taking it all too seriously – and then feeling certain that I needed medical help as soon as possible, but that no one would believe that unless I made a big deal about it myself. I had to begin by taking my own needs seriously instead of trying to ignore them.

Looking back, there were intuitive hints for years: there were dreams of trying to pull some kind of sickening white stuff out of my mouth – it just kept coming and coming; I needed to get it out of my body. There were many dreams of becoming too crippled to walk, my feet not having any power or coordination. The moment I finally landed into full body "knowing" that my body was truly very sick was after telling my (very intuitive) friend about what I thought might be happening. "What can I do to help?" She asked.

That's when I knew. Something undeniable slipped into place. It was a feeling of acknowledgement, of resonance, of coming into focus. I no longer felt foolish or confused. At last I surrendered to being honest with myself, come what may.

My friend gave me Reiki treatments once a week for several months. In one session, before I shared my "white fluff" dreams, she had a vision that she was pulling some kind of white "stuffing" out of my abdomen. Another time she shared a vision of icebergs melting, and as they were melting I was getting better. I took that as a positive sign. My immune system was not functioning well, and I felt cold all the time. 96.4 was my "normal"; 98.6 felt like a running a fever, with sweating and an erratically racing heart. The image of melting ice also connected with the idea that my life force had been "stuck in deep freeze" for a long time. Now that I've gotten back into painting and writing it feels as if this frozen potential is flowing again. After many years of feeling stuck and confused, I'm now finding it easier than ever to sense and trust intuitive guidance and then act accordingly.

7. Permanent Records

This piece began as a charcoal sketch done in Jungian therapy in early 2009, before I knew about Lyme. Starting therapy that winter was my first attempt in many years to reach out for help in searching for answers and to confide about my private storms. This sketch depicted the disintegration of so many of the "official" aspects of my identity. Some papers represented certificates of special career training and diplomas that had once seemed important, but now seemed to make no difference in my ability to make a living, advance along a career path, or experience well-being – they had become mere slips of paper. Other papers represented legal documents and contracts: all my former jobs, an expired teaching license, two marriage licenses, two sets of divorce papers. It seemed as if most of what used to define "me" had been "blown away."

Soon after sketching this piece, I began to learn about Lyme disease and to identify with anecdotes about other people's experiences of it. This inspired me to search through boxes of my old journals (there was a closet-full). There I discovered descriptions bearing witness to this illness and its effects. It was amazing to have a whole new lens through which to view past struggles. The new "Lyme colored lens" put such a different spin on everything. This process of review and revision helped me begin to release a cache of long hidden

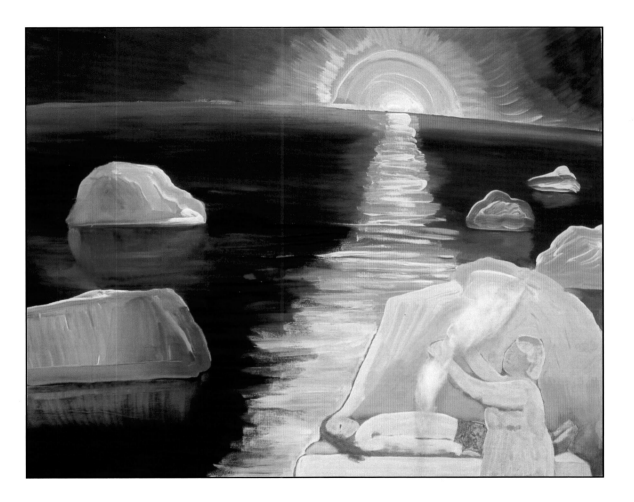

6. Fluff and Icebergs,
acrylic and cotton on birch
16" x 20", 2010

guilt, anger, shame, frustration, and resentment. Assembling sections from those journals suddenly became a compelling project. Finally I began to connect the dots of all aspects of my experience, inner and outer, and to acknowledge the body's need for more attention and support. Those notes, describing changes in my health and abilities, became the foundation for three hours' worth of health history interviews with my new doctor. Having these details in writing was essential for me because within the flow of a spoken dialogue I was often unable to recall important facts or to speak articulately. I would stammer nervously, loose my train of thought, and sweat profusely when trying to focus and give clear answers. I was what is informally called "a mess."

Later that year, as leaves began to fall, I felt drawn to release the past symbolically by burning much of my old writing. The empty clip on this painting is an artifact of that purge. Suspended from it hang three pages of journal entries from four months in 2002. They describe the dramatic fluctuations between sickness and health that can be common with chronic Lyme disease and its attendant co-infections.

LYME LOG FROM JOURNALS

8-6-02 "This a.m. my head and body ache. ...Looking back [on the past school year and setting intentions for more self care in upcoming year when I would teach grades 3-4] I now realize what I accepted as a "normal" day included awakening panic stricken, having to pray in order to get out of bed, dreading the day ahead, not knowing what to feed myself, not wanting to feed myself, putting on a good face and clothes – hard, because I didn't know what to wear nor want to go out into public, exhausted, wrung out, sore all over, fragile, easily enraged or moved to tears. Little appetite nor centeredness to tune in about my needs. Came to tears or other strong emotions on a daily basis, and frequently had a hard time thinking quickly. Frequent colds and sore throats. Hard time sleeping, frequent anxiety attacks on personal time."

8-14-02 "Why does the bottom keep dropping out? Between 10 pm when I lay down, and 11 pm, I went from fully focused, positive, confidant, relaxed, to feeling psychologically hazed, deranged, caught off-guard, like I was living a nightmare. That's the typical pattern. I can't figure out how it falls apart, what my part is..."

[undated, middle of August] "Hot flashes, aching body and heart, tears... Many moments I almost feel I could capsize, but I keep going. ...My conception of TIME changes radically from hour to hour...100's of times today I felt like giving up. Some glandular swelling, some toxic release left..."

[undated, end of August] "Restful sleep, peaceful and calm awakening, inner harmony, sweet gladness about the day, the future, seeing with heart open. I feel more balanced, centered and whole than almost ever in recent memory. I feel more settled and stable

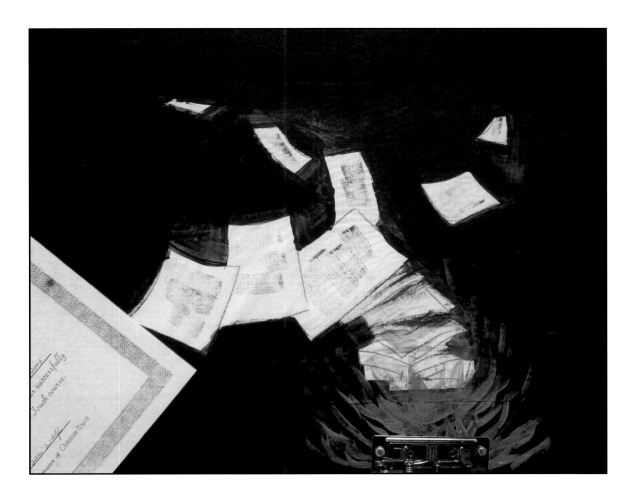

7. Permanent Records
charcoal, acrylic, paper, string, and metal on art board
16" x 20", 2009

than in a long time, and that it is really who I am. I do not believe I am manic depressive. I believe I have been living with intense inner change, also grief. I have been sad. These days are so bright. Since Tuesday I've felt like I've been in a new life – good vibes, inner strength. I'm excited about school starting."

9-6-02 "Things went very well at school this week in my class. It is alive – I love having a bigger class. LOTS of joy!!!"

9-12-02 "...angry and cried uncontrollably, so upset at recess that I couldn't stand it and cried. Blurry boundaries – I feel all worn out and mixed up. Period." "I don't feel strong and confident. Back to feeling very vulnerable and childlike and like I can't maintain a sensation inside of being grown up. Weary. Where is my health? Feels like my whole body is aching, shoulders and neck and face – all stiff and yucky, joints sore. I feel contaminated. I don't know where the feelings of being enthusiastic and positive and mature went to. It feels like being a different person. I feel like I'm dreaming. I feel very introverted. I am disgusted by these fluctuations and exhausted by trying to be certain ways. I feel like my life is so messed up, it's hard to know what to do. Clarity disintegrates so quickly. I forget who I am so easily. I feel numb and sore and exhausted. Can't find perspective through mental effort. Can't make myself be happy or content. I feel confused – strained mentally, emotionally, physically." "Nothing is making sense. It all seems random and I have no enthusiasm or conviction. It feels like I'm in a dream and I can't wake up and no one is coming to help – it all seems senseless."

9-20-02 [nice printing again] "Another delicious week of hard work and enjoying it, at school. I am glad to work there. I am glad to be that role. Living abundantly, counting blessings. Flowing into Friday

again, a quick week. Living deeply each day, connected, full, but not too much... Relishing life. Appetite for food and life."

10-2-02 "Head buzzing. I have a hard time letting go of mental control mode – like getting stuck in the "on" position. No emotions, frozen. Not caring to be with others or do things for pleasure. Overwhelmed. I feel like there's a thick dark wall between me and the world, like my eyes can't see the colors."

10-3-02 "I'm sad and mad and exhausted and unhinged. ...I feel I am in a world in the fog, in my own universe."

10-4-02 "A lot of energy in my pelvis and R hip joint and heart. Right now I feel warm, relaxed, present. Coming out of almost a week of feeling unbalanced, anxious, tense, afraid, worried, blustery, angry, sad, confused. My moods were so strong and charged so much this week and I went in and out so quickly. I am getting bored with my own stories, how things are always so complex and on the edge and up for questioning and uncertain and complicated with contorted conflicts. It would be a blessing to go on in a much simpler way... to not be delusional and lost in the nightmare quality of life... The forces effecting my moods and perceptions feel enormous. I have no way to control or challenge them mentally. I can only keep surrendering."

10-8-02 "Tuesday. Disconnected to past – unhinged. Paintings, memories of teaching... I seem to be standing on the outside looking in, estranged from life flow. Disconcerting – can't find warmth in the present. Sub-level not surface-level emotions. Like a radio on inside but can't hear it on the outside."

10-9-02 [after massage] "Feeling more calm and relaxed than in a long time... I feel very glad and excited to be teaching again."

10-11-02 "Will I ever stop feeling like I'm going insane, periodically? Will it get worse? I am terrified of flaking out. Will I ever learn to manage my stress better? Will I feel more emotionally stable? Are things as crazy as they seem? I am so tired. I am tired and I want to go home."

Friday [no date] "More possible chicken pox. [Several students in my class have chicken pox] Enjoying sleep (when I can — still up at 2:30, hard to go under again.) Actually everything seems to have a dreamlike quality, as if my senses and feelings were muted."

10-12-02 "Weird perceptions. Chicken pox [or shingles or other unknown rash] emerging, little "fly bites" itchy. Arthritis ache in right arm. Noises loud, can't understand how I got here. Sensitive all over. I am sick. Outgassing poisons through the skin. It feels like I'm in a dream, nothing is clear. It feels like someone else did those paintings. I can't find myself – the self who can do that. I feel lost to myself and not sure how to get back or go forward. I'm sick and tired of running into one rut after another. How the hell am I supposed to trust ANYTHING if the things I feel deeply don't last? I give up. I'm done. Take me home. I withdraw from this course..."

10-14-02 "Also I am aware that even when I am "out of sorts" lately, it is small rocking compared to a year ago. I feel more present and centered than in a long time."

10-18-02 "Itchy skin, It feels like I'm stuck inside a nightmare and I can't wake up. People not taking it seriously when I say I'm sick or exhausted. I want to quit."

Wed. "Every day different, very much. Contemplating leaving the school mid year if possible....last night I put great willpower into calming my body... Feeling strong, looking forward to next month of school." "Considerations: making transition out of this school. I have felt much anger and disgust and antipathy this month and heard myself saying same words as in marriage: 'I can't take this anymore, I want out.' Yet also slowing down and considering how I could do this departure differently. I really do love the children and the work."

10-25-02 "Tired irritated worn out disgusted, more rash – maybe shingles. I've Had it up to Here! Mtgs NON STOP 8-5 This is unsustainable."

10-29-02 Wed. "Intense headaches, some nausea ~ not cresting. Body not happy but soul and heart ~ intense week."

11-1-02 "It couldn't get much hotter than this. So much shit, my body is almost convulsing. Tail bone hurts, gut, neck, throat. I'm in deep heavy labor. Sore all over, emotionally as sore as can be. It is all coming to a head. I can't take any more intensity without exploding. Up until midnight 3 days in a row now. I hurt all over. I hurt so bad it feels like I'm being ripped apart or going to explode."

11-2-02 "This is really intense but I'm getting through it. After two days of hell, I am now more complete, stable, grounded. A lot of pressure in tail bone area."

11-5-02 "My pelvis aches."

"Sat. a.m. the tide has turned. Uplift! From grayest gloomy mood irritable, grouchy, to hopefulness and RELIEF!"

Sun. a.m. "I feel almost too tired to do anything. Fatigue radiating out of [picture of thymus gland on chest]. Thymus gland, heart area feels very strained. Like when you lose your breath and strain for air. I have another sore throat and sinus infection. I feel very vulnerable. I also feel relieved of the effort of trying to control. Letting go of the classroom and parent teacher conferences is one more huge release...my heart pulled me through this...I want to be all that I can be. I want to feel deeply fulfilled I want to wake up to the divine in daily life and not go back to sleep."

11-25-02 "Palpable stability coming in, up through my feet. Patchy fog, clearing."

Day after Thanksgiving – "Mind feels like scrambled eggs. No certainty."

8. Bar Code

For people who have had Lyme disease for a long time before starting treatment, it is not unusual to get a negative blood test. The blood tests are not perfect. The bacteria can live inside our cells, cloaking themselves in the cells' membranes, thereby disguising themselves from our own immune system. The body's immune system can give up fighting so there are no longer antibodies or "bullets in the streets" as signs of an active immune response in a "war" against an "invasion." In the absence of a positive blood test as proof of Lyme disease, I put together an extensive written health history from memories and journal entries to describe what was "normal," how that changed, and when. This not only provided clues to what the illness might be, it also turned up even more of an ants' nest.

The descent into the cavern I was currently in (2009) began in 2001, but during three hours of intense interviewing my Lyme-savvy doctor identified a probable "meeting with a tick" in 1984 when I was still in high school, and theorized that I might have been exposed much earlier in childhood. (I grew up in rural Northern Michigan, with dairy goats and deer in the woods and fields, and spent much of my free time playing and painting outside. Frequent respiratory and digestive ailments, fatigue, splitting headaches, and severely aching knees, legs, and ankles go back to early grade school. This was diagnosed as "allergies" for which I got weekly shots and "growing pains" for which I wore special orthopedic shoes to raise my arches.)

The possibility of having had Lyme changed my whole life story. "Amazing" is how I put it. "Coming out of denial" is how my doctor put it. Low energy, achy joints, swollen glands, loud popping sounds in the neck? "Normal," for this body. Other

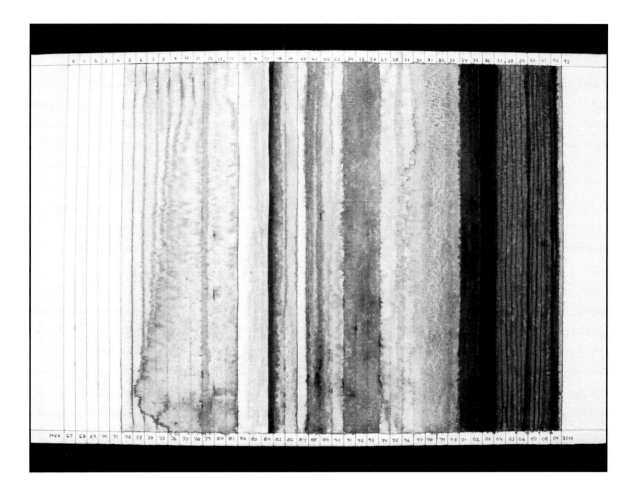

8. Bar Code
acrylic and pen on art board
16" x 20", 2010

conditions I had thought were "normal" turned out not to be; it's just that I'd been living with them for over half my life.

Curious to examine this history visually, I drew a column for each age/year of my life. As I began darkening patches to represent degrees of illness, I could see patterns forming; not only on the paper – a bar code sort of thing – but in terms of significant choices. I began to see how being sick in a Lyme-ish sort of way had affected choices I'd made in my social, educational, professional, and recreational life; based on my energy level, cognitive clarity, emotional stability – or the lack thereof.

9. Mad Math

This visual aid was inspired by the anti-drug campaign from the 1980's: your brain as an egg, a fried egg as "your brain on drugs." In recent years I often described my brain as feeling like "scrambled eggs" during those flipped-over-kayak times. My thoughts could easily get scrambled as well. When I imagined illustrating this, the idea of tangled yarn arose as a non-culinary alternative. Crocheting the healthy brain was a fun and healing experience; quite a "brain gym" workout as I stretched my concentration to 1) figure out how to make a brain from yarn in the first place, and 2) duplicate the hemispheres with some semblance of symmetry. The spiraled strands of yarn on the disc in the middle are supposed to be an enlarged view of the Lyme bacteria, a spirochete form. Anyone familiar may shudder at the close resemblance!

The background for the healthy brain is a piece of music I used to play at the Interlochen Arts Academy, an international school for the arts where I went to high school. In eleventh grade I was among the top students in the clarinet section. I was also a kid who liked to take standardized tests and typically came out several years above grade. That year, 1984, I was awarded the Rensselaer medal for Math and Science, along with a summer scholarship to the Rensselaer Polytechnic Institute as the top math and science student in the junior class. Instead, I chose to attend the Bennington July Program in southern Vermont and take classes in clarinet technique, music composition, and plant-based medicinal chemistry. The

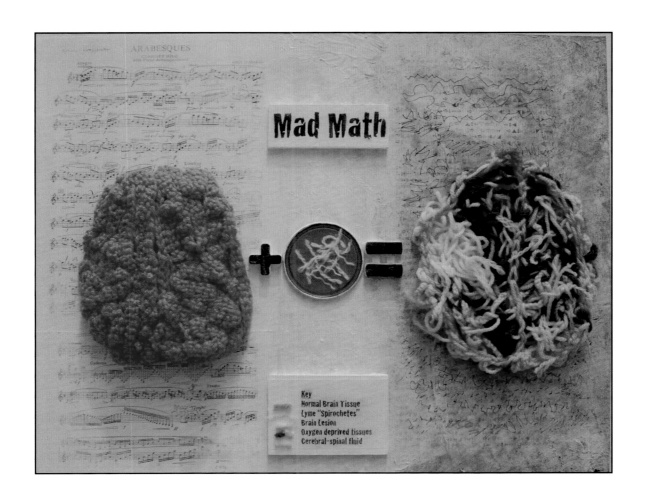

9. Mad Math
acrylic, yarn, paper, metal, and foam board on birch
16" x 20", 2010

rural Green Mountain scenery was a big draw. I loved to sit in the fields – writing, painting, thinking. I flourished in all my classes, and with faculty encouragement applied for early admission to the college. After joining my family for a vacation through scenic places down the East Coast from Mount Desert Island to Manhattan, I came home to discover that I had been accepted to Bennington for the fall. My plan was to double-major in Pre-Med and music composition.

Then, in late August, I came down with what felt like a case of the flu, feeling achy, feverish, and generally sick all over. This seemed to resolve except that soon I also felt as if my brain were being "rewired." It was a visceral, electrical sensation, with mental and emotional ramifications. For several reasons I decided to finish high school at Interlochen, much closer to home. In my journals from senior year the handwriting changes radically from the previously steady script of springtime. I describe trembling hands and intense energy in my spine as well as unshakable fatigue and roving aches and pains. I describe feeling uncharacteristically paranoid, anxious, tearful, depressed, hypersensitive, and mentally overwhelmed by jumbled thoughts, unable to focus without sheer effort. These episodes are contrasted by periods of feeling emotionally blank, numbed out, disoriented, "in another world," as if I am floating, dissociated from everything, as if my mind were too smooth and hard for any new fact to penetrate and stick. I wrote of being afraid of going insane. (And I never experimented with drugs or alcohol. Really.)

Reading text and music was a strain. I had already demonstrated a tendency toward dyslexia under pressure, but until that year I had thought of myself as a confident, dedicated, and very capable student. Following lectures became ever more difficult. Complex analysis of ideas under pressure, such as during essay exams, and committing new facts to memory became more difficult. I couldn't remember things well nor learn quickly anymore; it all became a huge effort. Instead of my usual two to three hours of practicing clarinet every day, I would often sit in the practice room zoning out, with the instrument on my lap, staring at the wall. At the beginning of the school year I still had the technical prowess to be a contender for an upper seat in the orchestra, but by the end of the year I had fallen to second from the bottom of the clarinet section in the concert band. Being in music ensembles felt awful – the noise made me dizzy. I often felt out of breath but blamed this, as well as the atrophy of other abilities, on my lack of practice. I couldn't understand why I seemed to be slipping in all subjects. I felt frustrated, embarrassed, awkward, and most of all guilty, as if I were failing to "get my act together," and therefore I tried to hide the problems even more. Some people thought I just had an attitude problem; a condition called "Senioritus." It became apparent to my (new that year) clarinet teacher that doing the required Senior Recital would be impossible for me, so I played one simple duet in another girl's recital instead.

The next fall I started college at Amherst, found the pace very daunting, and mid sophomore year I transferred to College of the Atlantic where I had more one-to-one help from teachers and was able to do more self-directed projects at my own pace. I never returned to the formal study of music, took only one required science class (squeaked by with a C), and somehow managed to never take a college level math class! I don't know if there are really any lesions on my brain, but working with numbers (even adding simple numbers) still doesn't come easily and I often make mistakes.

10. Strength as Weakness

How did these changes in ability not raise eyebrows? For one thing, most people close to me already knew I loved the humanities and visual arts as much as music, math, and science, so the switch to art, religion, and philosophy courses at Amherst, and then to philosophy and education at COA were still "within my profile" of interest. Also, since I didn't believe that taking a "time out" to collapse was possible, I just kept using whichever foot worked better. While memorizing and recalling data and facts became more difficult, pondering philosophical thoughts and writing my own ideas still came relatively easily. Perfectionism and pride as much as patience drove me to spend as much time and effort as necessary to complete assignments, so my grades remained "fine." No longer straight A's, but still looking "normal" with some B's and C's. It was frustrating to try so hard but not always excel.

Mentally and physically my health did improve somewhat after high school. If I did have Lyme back then, it may have been tamped down by antibiotics taken for other ailments such as sinus infections. Back then it was easy to get antibiotics. When I was younger my mother could even call the doctor, describe symptoms, and get a prescription filled for my dad to pick up on his way home from work! However, by the time I became a parent in 1995 at age 28, pediatricians counseled that it was wiser to try everything else before going the route of antibiotics – and I agreed. This change in climate of opinion set the tone for my refraining from seeking a doctor's help or medication to help with my symptoms later on; I was used to making the best of what I was going through on my own.

Looking back I have been recalling more and more episodes of illness in my 20's and 30's that might have been Lyme related: summer fevers with internally originating aches, pains, and fatigue (not due to any obvious overactivity such as sports). Sleeping and resting didn't make them go away. There were mysterious periods of searing pain in the torso. Once it was so severe that I went to the ER suspecting a heart attack, but no

cause appeared. "Probably a virus." "It must be a virus" was code for "there's nothing we can do for you," so when these pains came back I just endured them. Sometimes I could hardly move or breathe, the pains were so sharp. To stand up I'd have to roll over and crawl out of bed. I wondered how I could have strained and injured myself in my sleep. There were muscle aches and joint aches to the point where I'd be limping, but I always had some explanation: it was the bicycle ride, gardening, climbing stairs with laundry from the basement, standing up or getting out of bed without "limbering up" first. I was often very tired and "under the weather," but was able to push through it and keep working.

I used to believe that focusing outward and doing what was asked of me to the best of my ability was the definition of "acting responsibly." Eventually all this pushing and ignoring led to a rather robotic relationship to my work and other people. "Getting the job done" eclipsed a felt sense of connection with myself and other people. Now I am aware that I'm responsible for looking within and being honest with myself about what is going on inside as well. Sometimes that means

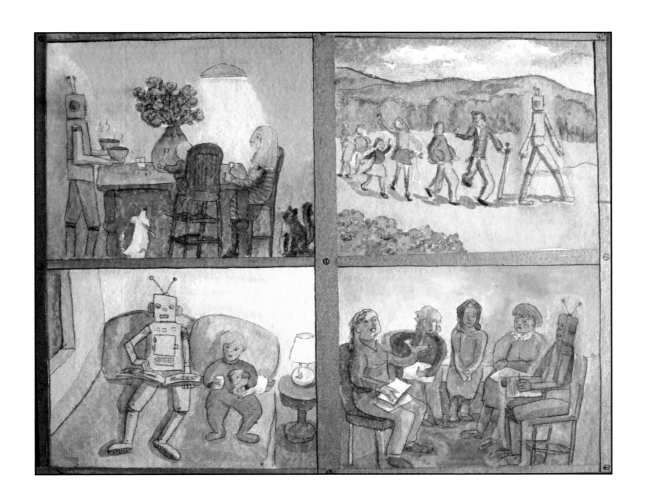

10. Strength as Weakness
acrylic and pencil on art board
16" x 20", 2010

asking for help. I'm discovering true strength can sometimes feel very soft.

11. Half an Apple

After college and a year and a half of international travel, I worked as a grade school teacher, moonlighting as a private art teacher and artist. My ability to concentrate and speak articulately was high enough to successfully manage complex jobs such as teaching in a one room school with 13 students (all grades, all subjects) and teaching K-8 art to 550 students a week (all of whom I knew by name and connected with as individuals), but I always felt the need to ramp up into a hyper-vigilant state of being "on edge" because it took great effort to focus, remember, speak, and lead coherently. I most enjoyed teaching small adult art classes such as Creativity Recovery Workshops at home. Most mornings in my 20's I woke up feeling tired and achy, but I adored my students and felt successful, even if teaching took all the effort I could muster. As with college, it seemed to me as if most other young adults around me had much more energy to spend in their off hours.

While friends, peers, and colleagues went out on the town, ran marathons, backpacked through mountains, and sought advanced degrees, I took only the minimum required "professional development" workshops and preferred to spend my limited free time quietly painting, writing, and reading on my own. Pregnancy and the birth of my daughter at the end of my 20's was a great excuse to take a time-out from formal education and formal employment. I was able to be a full time mom in a supportive community environment. Although I was often tired and mildly ill, my life style was low-key. I didn't have to work to support myself and could hang out with the toddlers at the sandbox.

Between 2001 and 2003 everything started to fall apart again. I was newly divorced, teaching art and grades 2-4 at a private school. For a few days at a time I would feel like a capable adult: Teacher, Student-Teacher Supervisor, Faculty Chair, Board Member, Single Working Mom. Then, for no apparent reason, I would slip into an internal sensation of profound anxiety and confusion which I defined at the time as "immaturity." I also described (only in my journals) feeling like

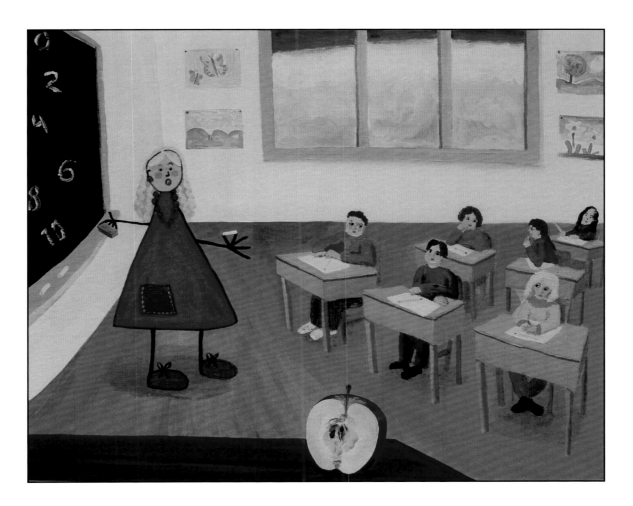

11. Half an Apple
acrylic on art board
16" x 20", 2009

a two dimensional "paper" person. Sometimes it felt as if I were physically floating in the air. Sometimes my legs ached so badly I had to pull myself up the stairs by the railing. Although I had so many other physical symptoms as well – a stiff neck, weird electrical sensations in my head and limbs, roving aches, odd rashes, and swelling in the joints – I viewed them each as a separate issue and chalked them up to "stress", "inevitable middle age aches and pains", "allergic reactions to eating nightshades" (potatoes and tomatoes), and "an allergy to poison ivy" (which I seemed to mysteriously be getting rashes from even though I knew to avoid the plants).

As in high school, I focused on appearing competent, hiding my symptoms, and interpreting my problems as signs of personal weakness. Unknown to me at the time, several students and a colleague of mine came down with Lyme disease, and all of them believe their exposure was on our school grounds; a forest with many deer. (Some were first diagnosed with arthritis, fibromyalgia, chronic fatigue, and depression before their true illness was determined and effectively treated.)

This painting portrays how I felt when teaching under the influence of a neurological state commonly described by Lyme patients as "brain fog," symbolized in the painting as an approaching bank of clouds or fog. The teacher is represented as a stick figure a child might draw. Although she is made up to be as "perfect" as can be in her color-coordinated outfit, students are beginning to suspect that she is "not all there." Like the numbers on the board there is still a degree of sensibility and order, but how it is being delivered is starting to seem somewhat floaty and tipsy. Teaching the Waldorf grade school curriculum involved much oral story telling and reciting of memorized verses and facts. Memorizing was futile for me, so I often felt like I was faking my way as a Waldorf teacher by using cue cards. I played up my strengths such as organizing the room and featuring student artwork so that anyone who entered saw orderliness and beauty.

In spring 2002, I declined the renewal of my contract. Over the summer my health improved enough that I reapplied for my old position and was re-hired, but by November I became too ill to teach and resigned. It seems hard to believe now, but at the time it didn't occur to me to share with anyone the difficulties I was facing. I was still operating from the perspective that I had somehow failed to maintain good health and was guilty of giving up; I'd failed to marshal the strength and balance to overcome my difficulties. Nor did it occur to me to apply for Disability or other formal support. I thought that was for people with a permanent impairment such as blindness. Without a job, I no longer had health insurance nor income to pay for expensive checkups out-of-pocket, so I didn't go to a doctor. Instead, I tried to treat some symptoms on my own with health food store items such as flower essences, herbal tinctures, and homeopathic remedies. I knew Reiki and other hands-on healing techniques that I could exchange with other practitioners for free, and I bartered a friend for Integrated Awareness sessions. While these holistic approaches did help sooth me somewhat, I continued to go through ups and downs, and overall there was the feeling of an undertow pulling me into deeper waters.

Looking back with more information, I now believe that the "brain fog" was most likely encephalitis and meningitis –

inflammation of the brain and membranes around the brain and spinal cord – a state beyond my ability to control any more than the teacher and class can control the weather outside their windows.

In this painting it was fun to mix different levels of abstraction and realism, including a perspective that is somewhat skewed and half an apple going brown. Another visual pun in this painting is that the three planes of the room converge behind the teacher. I did that on purpose to put the visual emphasis on her, but later realized that she is literally "in the zone of the vanishing point." Another joke, which I did intend, is that everyone has an eraser. Waldorf students are not usually given erasers (to promote best effort and concentration the first time around and avoid obsessive erasing and trying over). I gave everyone an eraser so that whatever was done could be undone if necessary; a positive spin on the idea of forgetting and an allusion to recovery.

12. Remember?

When looking for fonts to print this dialogue I stumbled across "School House Printed" and was tickled by the connotation of a school kid writing on the chalk board as a punishment. This explicit reference to "being guilty" made me laugh and confront the idea with humor: Was I really trying to be a space cadet? No. I made this painting soon after starting antibiotics in summer 2009. I was just beginning to realize that much of my short and long term memory loss could be given a new explanation that left all parties blameless. I used to think of myself as a "sharp" competent person, but more and more I felt frustrated about forgetting things – particularly verbal requests. "In one ear and out the other" had become the usual way of it.

One might think that taking notes would help, but trying to switch from listening to writing was as difficult as trying to translate words into another language. Before the Lyme diagnosis I usually blamed these listening and memory problems on being stressed out and preoccupied. As the situation got worse between 2001 and 2009, I lost all confidence to work outside my home except for a little cleaning and light gardening, both of which sapped my energy, but they could be done privately – little human interaction was needed, nor was reading or writing or math. I often felt childlike or simple-minded among other adults. I had difficulty following complex instructions, such as how to program the sprinkler system at the nursery where I watered plants.

At home I did some illustration work and enjoyed teaching private art classes to small groups of adults and children around my dining room table, but teaching just one class per day was exhausting. By 2008 I started to mix up students' names and felt too awkward facilitating discussions with the adults to continue even these intimate home-based classes. It was as if I were on autopilot. I just wanted to be alone and rest. I stopped offering classes and began passing-on my vast collection of art supplies to other teachers and home schooling parents – folding up camp. The one benefit of earning so little and spending so much of my savings to make ends meet was that I finally qualified for basic subsidized state health insurance. But I still didn't go to a doctor. I still took my

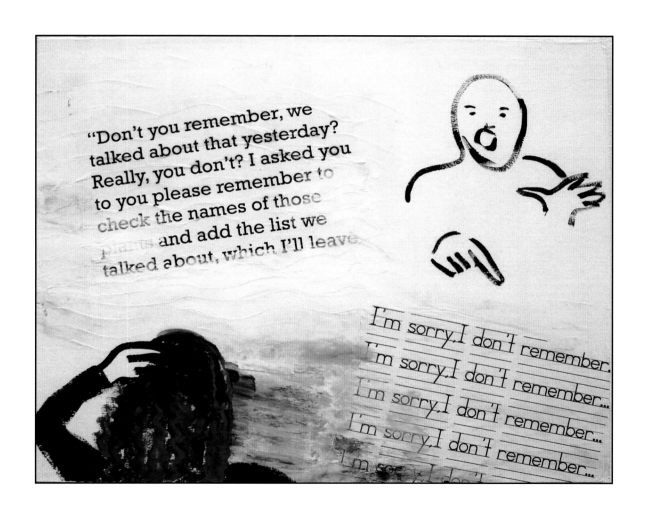

12. Remember?
acrylic on art board
16" x 20", 2009

challenges personally, as if I were to blame for being weak, and then I would also look outward and blame my single-parent/head-of-household/low income status for the stress.

Word finding was another challenge which affected my ability to engage in ordinary dialogue. In short spontaneous conversations, such as with drive-through tellers at the bank and clerks at the grocery store, I would often get stuck trying to remember simple words, fumble mid-sentence, and eventually I stopped trying. Any outings into the world – the library, bank, and grocery store (that's what it was down to) – were an enormous challenge. I would use breathing to control my high anxiety and just try to get the chores done and get home. I was mostly out of contact with all but two friends, rarely spoke on the phone with relatives, and used email instead. My verbal interactions with people were often "brittle" and short. My daughter got used to finishing sentences for me. "Honey, can you... um,...get me...that...um,...thing...?" "Your cup of tea?" "Yes, thanks!" Even friendly conversation required laborious effort. The best way to have a conversation was one-to-one with no distractions so that the other person could give me their fullest attention and thus be patient as I fished for words. A rare hour of "tea and talk" would totally wear me out, and yet those special times were the only times I really felt connected with the world outside my home. Friends didn't realize how difficult it was (or maybe if they did notice something, they just thought I was tense or in a hurry to go – because I was, trying so hard to sound normal.) If conversations were about familiar subjects, such as discussing spirituality and education with my friend Sue, it was easier to "get in the groove" and access that specific realm of vocabulary.

One day in the summer of 2009, one month into taking 400 mg per day of the antibiotic Doxycycline Hyclate, I enjoyed three personal, flowing, spontaneous, genuine, neighborly conversations with people in the grocery store! It was amazing! I was elated and grinning! It felt as if I were coming home from having been far, far away for a very long time. My doctor says I'm like a different person now. Currently I tutor one student a week and we're both enjoying it. I still make some silly mistakes but we can laugh about it.

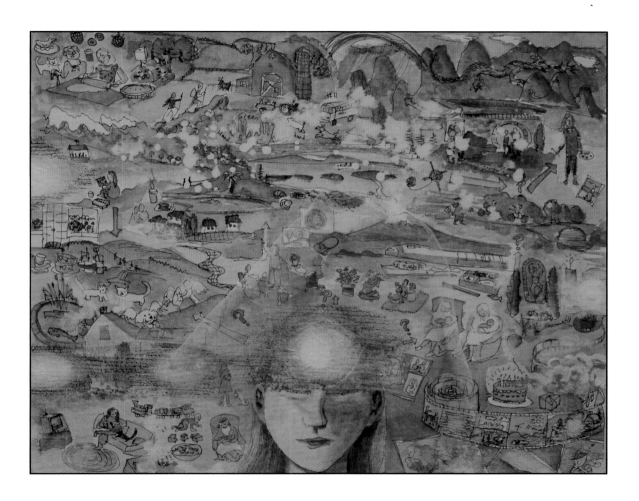

13. Brain Fog
acrylic and tulle on art board
16" x 20", 2010

13. Brain Fog

This painting portrays more properties of "brain fog." The images are all scenes from my past, so obviously I could remember them. Memories do not seem to become totally lost, but rather temporarily obscured, as if behind a veil. To put it another way, it is as if the "Files" still exist but the "Search/Find" command has been impaired. When asked to recall something in particular, on the spot, such as my son's birth date, it may be impossible to "get there" as fast as I need to. "Blanking out" is another way to describe it. I have forgotten my own phone number while in the process of dialing home. A difficulty I often faced while typing up my health notes was that I would "Select" a paragraph, "Cut" it, go to "Paste" it, and then forget where I was intending to put it. I'd have to put it back and retrace the whole thought process. Some periods were easier, but overall I was in a state of decline from 2001 to 2009. The "descent into becoming stupider" is what it felt like. In conversations I often asked people, "Have I told you this already?" having no certainty of the content of our recent conversations nor a clear memory of the order of contacts I

had made. Another quality of "brain fog" is when one is trying to focus on imagining an image, such as following a guided meditation or listening to directions about where to drive. Sometimes the inner mind-screen cannot hold an important image steady to build upon it, or it can appear like a blank, static TV screen which holds no images at all. Sometimes random images flutter by so fast it's as if a hyper toddler or monkey were holding a video camera.

Now, when I am well rested, my memory works much better. I often find it easy to generate and edit my own creative writing. I'm learning to be more amused than concerned when files "go missing" – or the bag of frozen corn, which I recently found "filed" in the cabinet by the cat food instead of in the near-by freezer. I'm learning to be more aware of the "present moment" and trust that what I really need to know is what I do know right now. Sometimes the blank-mind state seems like a "free trial sample" of what some people may meditate for years to attain. Paradoxically, this messed-up-mind thing has not been all bad: it's gotten me to reflect upon who and what I really am.

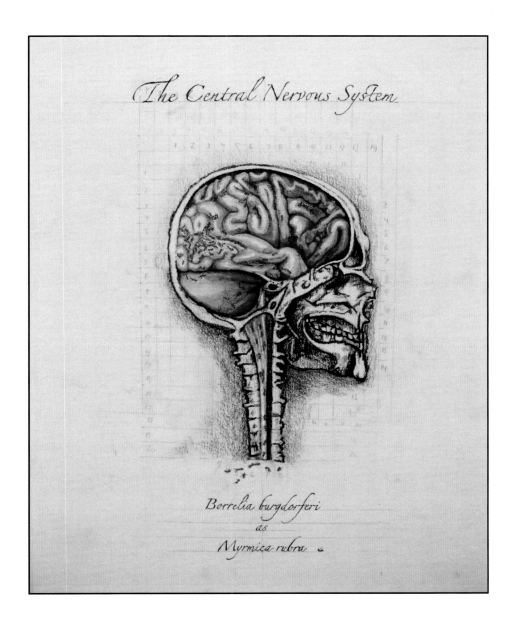

14. The Central Nervous System
pencil and acrylic on art board
16" x 20", 2010

14. The Central Nervous System

I admit that part of what inspired me to make this painting was my Lyme doctor saying, "Don't even try to get people to understand. Unless they've been through this, they just won't get it." Oh, what better challenge does the wounded-inner-child-as-artist need to incite her to try?

I started sketching from a photograph of Leonardo da Vinci's skull studies. The grid of numbers is a remnant of the process of doubling the size of the image. Leaving it in place seemed to add to the aura of a "scientific specimen," giving the ants even more of an invasive effect. (No matter how much we quantify and analyze our biological elements they continue to elude our attempts to fully control what happens to them.) The font, Cochin, appears elegant and old fashioned as if written with a quill. In the process of transferring the writing using carbon paper, it got a bit of a wiggle that adds a "nervous" effect. It also reminds me of letters written by elderly relatives whose penmanship was elegant but is starting to reveal the atrophy of fine motor control – another Lyme symptom I experienced when my hands would get tremors. The idea of ants to represent Lyme bacteria had been with me for a long time – from journal entries trying to describe periods of cerebral irritation. "Ants in your pants" is a common metaphor. The stinging red ants everyone in my community would recognize seemed even more appropriate. Virtually every resident of Mount Desert Island has been through the visceral experience of being stung by a red ant, and knows how the stinging slowly resolves through an ebb and flow of lessening intensity but prolonged irritation. Only a cutaway view of the brain would show the areas of mine seeming to be most effected, but I wanted a very alive-looking brain so I showed it from the outside. I didn't research areas and functions until after making this painting. It was amusing to discover that the highest density of ants was painted on the Primary Visual Cortex. Therefore a visual pun and a fun experience loop was unintentionally created: as we view this painting, the primary part of our brain processing this image is the Primary Visual Cortex – so, in a way, it becomes a self-portrait of whoever views it. (Whether they get it or not!)

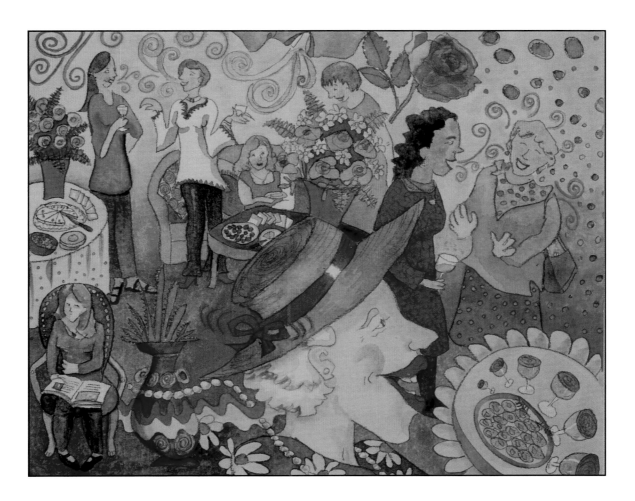

15. Party Pooper
acrylic and pencil on art board
16" x 20", 2010

15. Party Pooper

This painting began as a portrayal of "sensory overload." I wanted to depict the way I felt at a lovely luncheon several years ago which was the first big social event I had attempted in many months. As people gathered, the noise level rose, and the din of voices and colors made me feel overwhelmed, dizzy, and slightly nauseated. I felt like an anxious animal wanting to find a place in which to hide, and chose to focus on the vast collection of wonderful books in the host's house. As people came up to me offering conversation I felt small and meek. I had a difficult time focusing on what they were saying, and an even harder time thinking of something intelligent to reply. Stammering, shifty-eyed, I felt none of the mature poise I had possessed before the latest "Lyme Lowpoint." After that trial I decided (again) that I just wasn't up to socializing with groups any more, and so I avoided most gatherings until after starting medical treatment in summer 2009. Attending a party, concert, play, puppet show, poetry reading, or community supper was a once-in-a-long-while venture, sapping energy banked up by extra rest and usually followed by a day or more of "falling apart," including fatigue, high anxiety, irritability, headaches, and tearfulness. Sometimes when I drove to buy groceries I would stall in the parking lot, realize that I was going to be overwhelmed in the store, so I'd give up and drive home.

While there have been some significant improvements since then, I still feel "fragile" much of the time. I can become easily overstimulated, and am easily overwhelmed when I get tired. If I go to a public event or go out driving and doing errands for three hours I will soon feel tired, irritable, shaken-up, and sometimes experience the old tipsy and trembly feelings from a hypersensitive nervous system. Every day now includes some kind of soul-satisfying social interaction, usually via the telephone and internet, but my internal "battery" still seems to get drained quite quickly if I spend much time out in the world.

This painting, for me, has come to represent positive future possibilities. There is warmth and good food, animated discussion and laughter. The very air is coming alive with dancing ribbons and dots of music. I see it as a portrait of a buoyant celebration that I might enjoy someday.

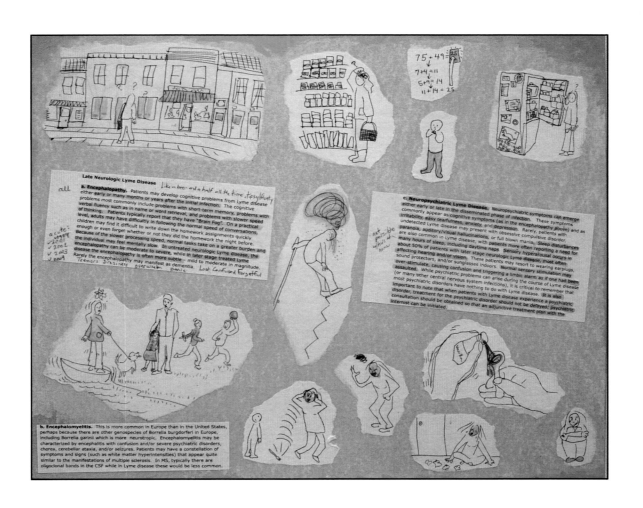

16. It's All in Your Head
acrylic, paper, pen, and highlighter pen on art board
16" x 20", 2010

16. It's All in Your Head

This panel illustrates some of the situations and conditions I frequently experienced due to the neurological symptoms of Lyme disease: On a small town main street, forgetting where the door was for a counseling appointment. Forgetting the counselor's name when asking a passerby for help (and I'd been there many times, including the week before). Spacing out while in the grocery store and looking in the refrigerator. "What was it I needed?" (Everybody spaces out sometimes, but this condition was daily.) Adding numbers mentally and not catching a ridiculous mistake. Becoming dizzy after climbing a short flight of stairs. Feeling tipsy all the time, as if slightly drunk, or as if I were in a little boat that was sloshing in little waves. Losing my temper over sharp sounds such as a fork hitting the floor, reacting out of proportion to the event as if I were being physically attacked. Trembling visibly when trying to do fine motor tasks such as pouring vanilla extract while baking. Frequently feeling traumatized out of proportion to what was happening, and then feeling scared of being so highly sensitive and emotionally vulnerable.

Ironically, my story is the reverse of most Lyme sagas. Many people who are sick with Lyme have gone through the experience of being told by at least one doctor (if not many) that their "illness" is "all in their heads." Even people with obviously debilitating physical symptoms have been told that they are making it up; role playing, manifesting psychosomatic symptoms, creating attention-getting dramas. My story plays a unique role in the emerging awareness of Lyme disease because I was the one trying to make it be "all in my head" for so long. I took all my symptoms personally. I believed that if I could only manage stress better and learn to maintain a more positive outlook on life – in other words, develop a more "mature and responsible attitude" – then the body would follow. I would be able to manifest health, wealth, long term loving relationships, a nice house, and all that. So I just kept focusing on correcting the imbalances I perceived to be within myself and blaming myself for not being able to "get my act together." I did this all in private. There was no attention-seeking through complaining about my symptoms. To the contrary, I didn't let my closest friends, family members, or my regular doctor in on the story. For years I feared I would risk everything if I let

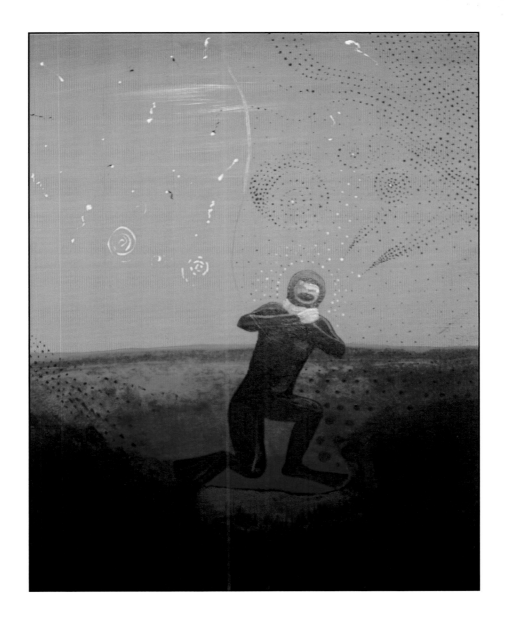

17. Asphyxiation
acrylic on art board
16" x 20", 2009

down my guard. I might lose my job, friends' patience, clients' respect, possibly even custody of my baby. I believed I needed to show the world that I could "hold it all together" on my own.

A paradox is that for most people with chronic Lyme, the disease is, quite literally, in their heads: swarming colonies of tunnel-drilling spiral-shaped bacteria are wreaking havoc with their brains. This isn't something any of us can cure by simply "cultivating a positive attitude."

17. Asphyxiation

Before making the association between my symptoms and an illness, I often described sensations in metaphorical terms, interpreting them as psychosomatic side effects of "personal issues." I told one therapist that I often felt panic stricken, and that sometimes for long periods of time I felt like a diver whose oxygen tank was empty or whose hose was blocked. Looking at that symbolically, I blamed stressful situations in my adult life and childhood, and examined where I was metaphorically

"stifling" myself through self-limiting beliefs. But no matter how much I "let myself feel the feelings," journaled, emoted, or "aired out my issues" through talking, I got no lasting relief. I just didn't seem able to "process" fast enough to "get ahead" in the game. Periodically, as symptoms would flair up, I would appeal for help from the invisible realm; "Beam me up, please, I can't breathe down here!" I felt trapped in my body and desperate for relief.

While all that purging and processing may have helped on some levels, it was a *Eureka* moment to read that colonies of Lyme bacteria and other tick-borne parasites would sap oxygen from the host body, particularly the brain. My body was, quite literally, becoming "oxygen starved." (I do still often look at life metaphorically, and want to credit my angelic guardians for listening to my appeals for help and for leading me to Pamela Weintraub's book about Lyme at the library. The cosmic message that came with that nudge was, "You've learned all that you can from this illness. Time to clean up the classroom.")

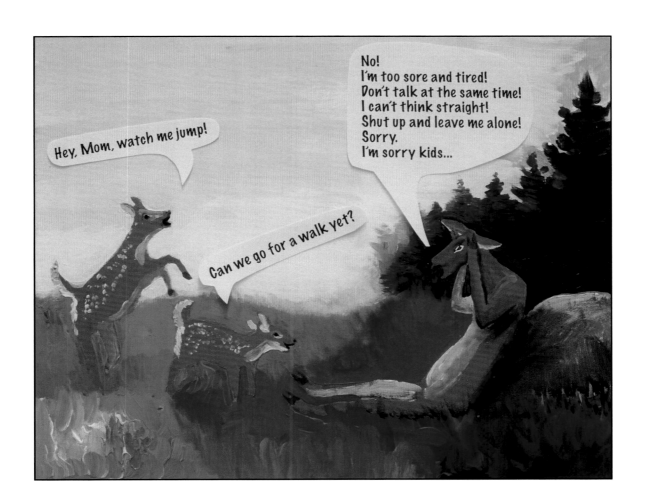

18. Poor Mother Deer
acrylic and paper on birch
16" x 20", 2010

18. Poor Mother Deer

The two people most affected by all this were my children. Looking back, we do share many sweet memories: sewing a beautiful quilt, cooking and art projects, in-depth studies on topics of their passionate interests. Overall, I'm glad to have been at home with them for so much of their childhoods. But there were many days that even simple tasks could overwhelm me. During "Lyme Lowpoints" I often felt breathless while reading aloud to my son. If he asked a question during the story, I might get irritated and weepy. Having to make the transition from focusing on the book to focusing on his question to finding my place in the book again was labor intensive! I often explained to my children that I was "stressed out" and needed to take a "time out" alone in my bedroom if possible. For several years I believed we were home schooling because it was what they needed, but looking back I admit it was also because I didn't feel capable, competent, or confident doing any work outside the house, and home schooling made me feel "respectfully employed." Compared to most other home schooling families we were very house bound. We almost never traveled or attended events with other people. For a while when my son was a toddler, I tried attending a parent/child play group but could barely think straight when there. The lights, sounds, and activity level made my head swirl. I felt dizzy, mute, anxious, and shy, and couldn't remember most people's names from one week to the next. Eventually we stopped going. "Barely coping" was passing for "normal"!

In spring 2009, before I learned about Lyme, I decided to enroll my children in public school for the fall, knowing I just didn't have the strength or mental ability to be a good home school teacher any longer. People started asking, "What are you going to do with all that free time – go back to work or school?" And I would think, "Sleep. Or die." There was no motivation to do anything else. It felt like my only motivation for staying in a body was to see my children grow up.

Once the treatment for Lyme was underway and my mind began clearing, I began to see the impact of my illness on my children. I began to solicit more professional support such as informing their teachers about the effects of Lyme. One of my

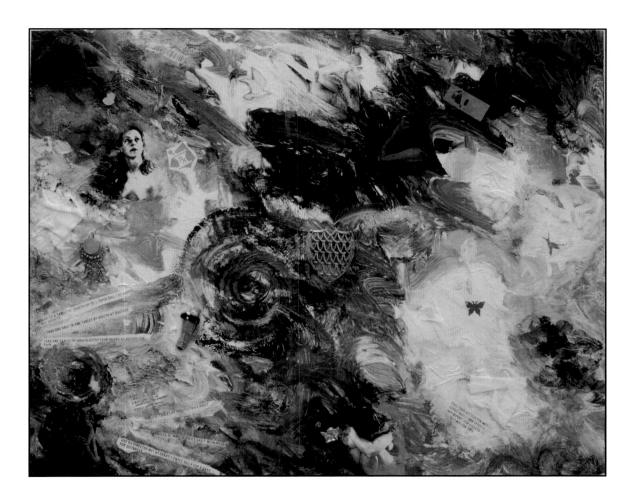

19. Fight/Flight
acrylic, paper, metal, cloth, plastic, and feather on art board
16" x 20", 2010

daughter's teachers asked her if she was aware of how often she finished other people's sentences. She laughed with me as we realized the conditioning she'd gotten from being around my "special needs" all day. At the recommendation of a friend I initiated contact with a social and health services agency which sent a case worker to make house calls. With her sympathetic and compassionate support I began to open up to even more help such as family counseling. It required huge courage for me to let people in to witness my private world and I felt very vulnerable when admitting I needed help. But the more I did, the more grateful I became to receive that support. Family counseling continues to support us in finding a new healthy normal.

The idea for this painting arrived one afternoon as I went for a walk in a cemetery near my home and saw deer tracks in the snow. I started thinking of all the deer with Lyme and that they might feel as badly as I did. Suddenly the cartoon image of a deer family came to mind and I bolted happily home to begin this painting. Every time I look at it I can't stop laughing. When it was hanging at the first gallery someone called me to report that the painting itself was "ticking." I checked. Sure enough! Perhaps there was an insect in the wood, who knows, but the painting really did make a rhythmic ticking noise!

19. Fight/Flight

In this painting I wanted to depict the incoherent storminess of feeling trapped by illness and yet struggling to find peace of mind and courage. I envisioned a painting with hurricane-like swirls of black and white with little colorful objects sticking out. I found the heart-shaped shield in a parking lot that morning as I walked my son to school. Then I discovered a little box of collage bits (gathered years before, for a different project) which all worked perfectly in this one! Expressing my inner struggle visually was incredibly uplifting. My willingness to trust inspiration increased because of the way this painting came together – it was healing to have such a coherent creative experience! This illustrates how healing can be experienced on the level of the mind, in spite of physical symptoms, and how being willing to look at what is most difficult can begin to transform it.

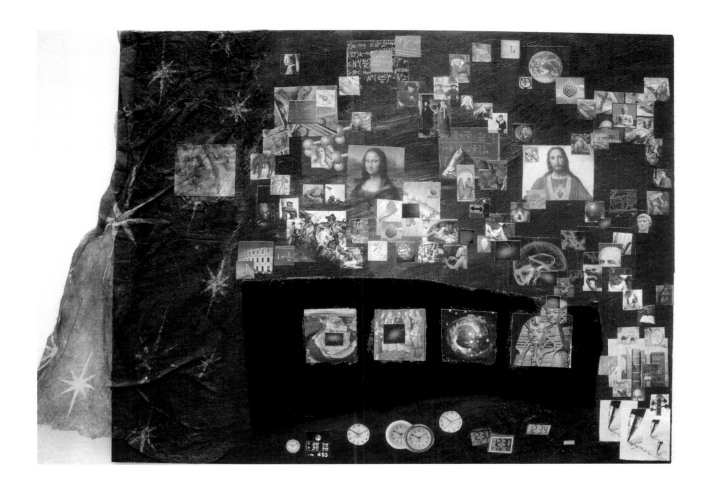

20. Insomnia
acrylic, cloth, and paper on art board
16" x 20", 2010

I wish that everyone recovering from any serious or chronic illness could talk about it with a counselor because trauma can accumulate just from being ill, and this trauma can also be released in many ways. I knew I needed help with this; I couldn't just take medicine to get better. Also, anxiety is one of the dominant symptoms of Lyme disease. One feels anxious even before there is a cause – it's as if a thumb is already pushing the fight/flight button. Neurotoxins from the bacteria in the brain may be one cause. Now that I have medicine to help with the physical symptoms, and now that I can speak articulately again, one-to-one counseling is a useful experience which supports me in reassessing my outlook on life. I can share what I've been through and revalue my life with a witness. My confidence is being bolstered. Now when I'm going through a neurological "rough patch" I'm more likely to remember that this body is highly sensitive and not to become self-critical or engage in any serious decision making. Sleep aids and anxiety medication have helped my body remember what "calm" is, so now I can "find this place on the dial" more easily on my own. The storms that come don't last as long.

20. Insomnia

Insomnia was the inspiration for the first painting I made in January 2010. Although my health had significantly improved, I still wasn't exactly feeling great. Daily household tasks and parenting were still taking most of my energy, and I was trying to fit in a daily nap if possible. I hadn't painted much since the initial burst of inspiration from summer. But the paints and brushes looked so enticing that I finally gave in and sat down. How can I paint when I'm still so sore and tired? I wondered. Suddenly, the vision came of a darkened room with tiny colored squares floating above a bed, representing the endless streams of thought that seem to flow when one is too tired to focus but too wired to drift off to sleep. Okay, I thought, that's a nice image. I can relate to that. But what about the colored squares? Magazine clippings? I didn't have any in the house, having jettisoned most of my collage supplies the previous summer. Then the mail came, and in the box was a catalog, full of little colorful squares with the most perfect images! Using a razor blade I cut out almost every one and by bedtime had finished the collage. Rather than overcoming symptoms in

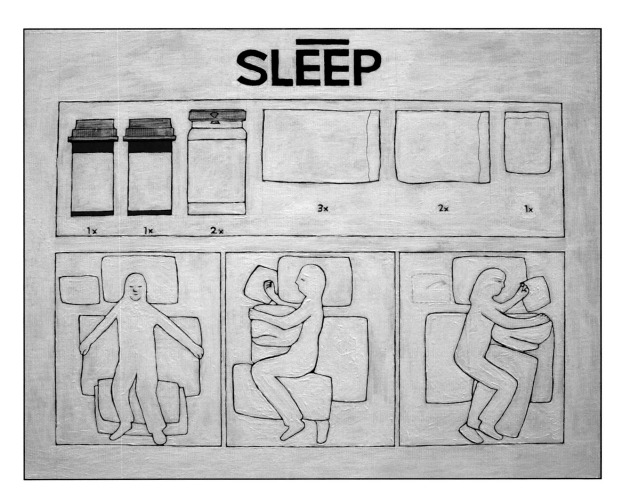

21. Sleep – Assembly Instructions
acrylic and permanent marker on birch
16" x 20", 2010

order to do art, art emerged as a way to honor the struggle. That got the momentum going. Within two months, all the other paintings for the exhibit had been completed.

21. Sleep – Assembly Instructions

During the initial health history interview I was asked if I used extra pillows at night. "Yes," I replied, thinking that was all. "How many? Where?" my new doctor prompted, looking serious. I had to stop and think. It was both amusing and gratifying to let someone in on those ridiculous facts of bedding down! It had become a nightly ceremony. It started with a body pillow when I was pregnant and over time I added four more pillows. Sleeping isn't simple, it's an installation project! It's a matter of proper placement and elevation of parts to reduce the strain on tender nerves and sore joints.

Having pillow combo and placement down to a science, my doctor and I began addressing the insomnia and pain management part of the scheme. In *The Power of Now* (2004) Eckhart Tolle recommends being present with pain instead of just trying to make it go away, and he explains that this awareness will help dissolve the "pain body." Sometimes I do that, at other times I take strong analgesics. I've come to accept a phrase I used to pooh-pooh, "better living through chemistry." Valerian tincture, lavender tea, Clonazepam, Advil, Extra Strength Tylenol – whatever it takes, I'm willing to give it a try! Sometimes one thing works for a while, then after a while it doesn't. Getting more sleep at night and resting more during the day have been essential to the healing process.

Now, over a year later, I still use all those pillows but the left side of my body is usually free of pain. Oddly, the right side, from head to toe, still ranges from slightly strained and numb to highly painful, raw, and "scraped," depending on how much activity I engage in, whether I'm fighting "what's going around," and how much rest I've gotten. Napping still feels out-of-character and rather lazy, but maybe that will change with more practice!

This painting was fun to make. The style was inspired by IKEA furniture assembly instructions. Creating it was a

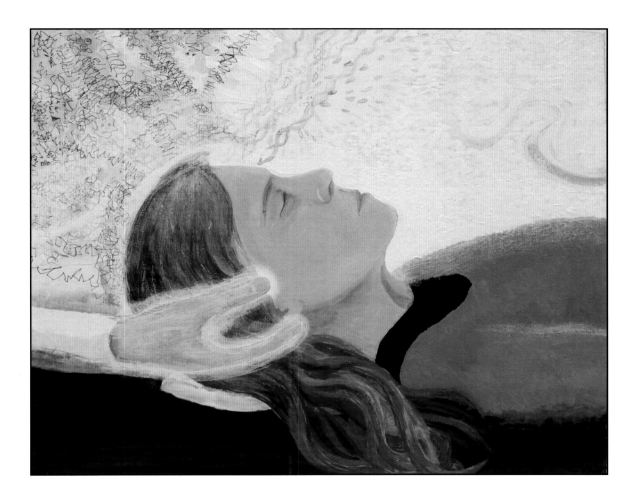

22. Helping Hands
acrylic on birch
16" x 20", 2010

therapeutic challenge. Sometimes my left hand was trembly, another neurological symptom. It could be steadied by holding the other end of the paintbrush with my right hand (I'm left-handed), or by bracing my hand on the paper. These tremors were not detectable when I used firm pressure, such as drawing in pen or making broad or rapid strokes of paint. They were most disruptive when I was trying to paint accurately into tiny corners. I listened to soothing piano music and worked in short segments with stretch breaks, meditatively painting over the whole image three times. Over the past year these tremors have largely subsided and only return during episodes of high stress, heightened nerve sensitivity, not getting enough rest, or in the midst of an additional immune challenge such as catching a cold – (which implies still having some periods of tremors daily or weekly, it's just not a constant condition).

22. Helping Hands

Therapeutic Massage, Reiki, Shiatsu, and CranioSacral Therapy have been very effective in helping me find inner calm and integrate so much change in the past year and a half. For three years, before learning about Lyme, I had considered going to an Osteopath who was helping some of my friends with spinal and cranial issues. Finally, as I was working on these paintings in early 2010, I got around to making an appointment. The D.O.'s subtle, noninvasive touch improved the flow of cerebral-spinal fluid around my brain which helped "dissolve" the feeling of "mental discombobulation." It was so affirming to hear that my private experience of inner mental and emotional turbulence had a detectable physiological counterpart! It was also interesting to be told that earlier treatments wouldn't have helped. There had been so much physical imbalance that I needed to have been on medications such as antibiotics first, for a while, before the nervous system was stable enough to make use of this kind of subtle energetic support. I said that perhaps that is why I hadn't come in before. "Yes, your body knew," the D.O. said. An image that came to me during that first session was that the damaged nervous system is like a cat that gets scared up a tree by a fierce barking dog (infections and trauma). Antibiotics are a dog catcher, and the Osteopath is a firefighter who is climbing a ladder to gently persuade the kitty that it's safe to come down

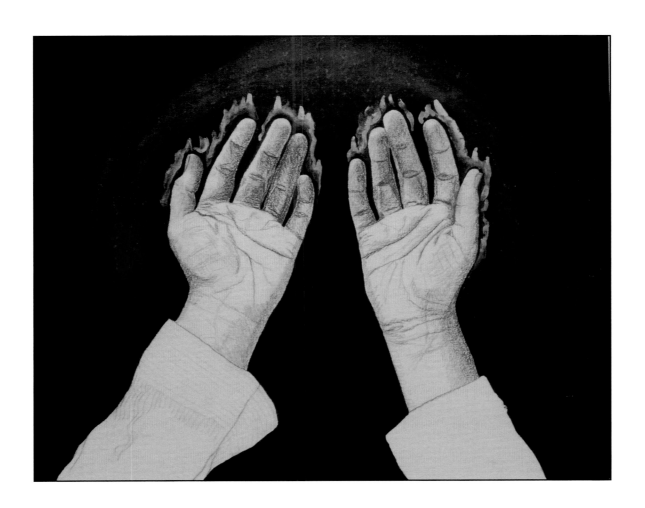

23. Side Effects
acrylic and pencil on art board
16" x 20", 2010

now. This painting is based on imagery that came to mind during my second session, involving many emotionally charged images and the acceptance of support for releasing them.

23. Side Effects

A common antibiotic for treating Lyme, Doxycycline Hyclate, makes one highly sensitive to sunlight. During the first week on it, I called the clinic to ask if it was normal to feel a sort of icy wind or mild burning sensation on my hands and was told yes, that was a possible side effect. Having a little boy and a part time summer gardening job, I couldn't exactly stay inside all day as advised, so I tried wearing sunblock. Until I read *The Lyme Disease Solution* by Kenneth B. Singleton M.D., M.P.H. (2008), chock full of self-help details, I didn't understand that sunblock wouldn't help. But by then my hands and face were badly burned. It took six months to fully recover, including growing new thumb nails. I invested in some soft, silky, sun-proof clothing including broad-brimmed hats and light weight gloves that I now wear every time I go out on a sunny day.

A second side effect of all the health challenges I've been through and all the methods of healing I've tried is that a lifetime worth of stifled anger has been burning away. Underneath the frozen layers of denial, grief, and depression lay a red hot lava layer of anger. With every step of physical healing I have found that there is an emotional counterpart of release, then a phase of reintegration.

A third side effect of being ill and dealing with a long period of treatment is that it induced me to seek solace and comfort beyond the (seemingly unattainable) physical level. I loved *The Disappearance of the Universe* by Gary Renard (2004), and *The Interior Castle* by St. Teresa of Avila, translated by Mirabi Starr (2003). Although St. Teresa lived five hundred years before me, her descriptions of her own health challenges and the spiritual transformations she was going through gave me much counsel and encouragement. Learning about the "Inquiry" process as described by teacher Byron Katie has also played a key role in how I deal with anger and fear, particularly regarding the future of my health. It has been comforting to have models of how to look at life differently, which support me

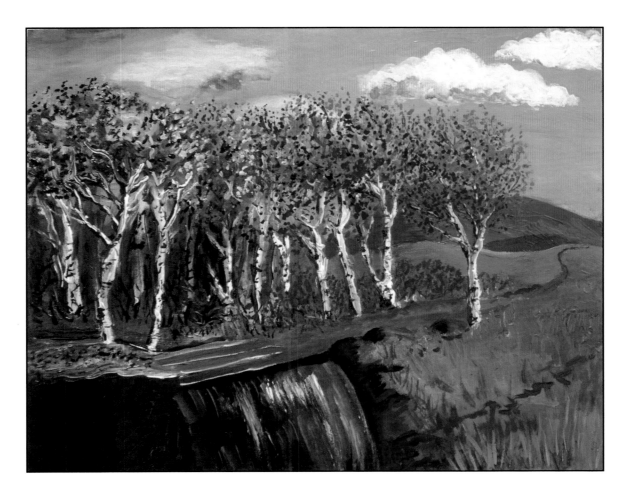

24. Path of Recovery
acrylic on art board
16" x 20", 2010

in accepting what I am going through at the same time as I'm finding the courage to make changes in my life and ask for help.

A fourth side effect of entering the healing process is that my life has been "lit" from within; I'm learning to trust intuition and inspiration more than ever before. I've been "on fire" with enthusiasm to be creative and to communicate. This painting was fun to have lying around the studio; the open hands kept receiving all manner of objects.

24. Path of Recovery

When I get very run down, all the color goes out of life; everything seems dull, devoid of vitality and meaning. I feel no emotional connection with anything or anyone, even my children. Before I began treatment for Lyme, this state had become the norm. I could act happy to be polite but those feelings weren't really there. Looking back I now interpret it as the immune system being overwhelmed and trying to send me the signal to stop trying to distract myself and get down to business and attend to the "state of emergency." There simply was no extra fuel for anything but surviving.

The summer I began treatment, I began to experience random breakthroughs into vitality and well being, which literally seemed to bring more color to daily life. I began enjoying and taking pleasure in seeing nature's colors, quite literally. From a couple of random hours per week in the beginning, to several hours at a time several days per week, my life increased in color and vitality.

As my mind cleared more and more, I engaged more with the world around me. There was still physical pain, but month by month there were significant improvements. I kept a daily chart of symptoms, so it might be that on a scale from 1-10 the pain was a "5" instead of an "8." In the beginning, any amount of exercise, such as walking around the block, could leave me hobbling. After a while the inflammation was reduced so that more days than not I could take a longer walk, enjoy it, and feel refreshed instead of drained. My hands and arms no longer ached constantly.

Even after months of treatment, common symptoms were mild to severe arthritis, mild nausea, temperature swings, sore muscles, achy joints and achy bones, pressure in the spine and head, and random nerve pain. But compared with before treatment, it was the difference between being so sick as to not even want a body, to rediscovering an interest in life and having a sense of curiosity about the future, even if feeling ill.

About five seasons into treatment I experienced nearly three pain-free weeks for the first time in years! I was able to swim and hike without paying for it later. That wonderful taste of having a body which was simply a vehicle for relishing life did not endure, but it was a window into the possibility of what could lie ahead.

Now, a year and a half into treatment, I would describe my body as having a "fragile state of health" that is easily upended by stress or exposure to common illnesses. If I overdo it, such as a three hour drive around town doing chores, that day and the next I become easily flustered and irritable, hypersensitive to touch, light, and sound, my skull and the base and top of my spine become sore, and my whole right side starts to feel irritated and strained. If stress continues and I cannot stop to lie down and rest right away, that strained feeling becomes a raw, scraped, burning sensation from head to toe. Little infections may still last for weeks. So I continue to live a very low-key life style compared with most people my age, staying at home reading, writing, and resting while my children are in school. But I am radiantly and creatively engaged in life again. My emotional and mental stability is more reliable; as long as I'm not too tired I'm able to think clearly and communicate in the moment most of the time, in a way that feels intelligent and "tuned in." Cranial irritation and headaches may be persistent, but they have become less severe. Friends of mine with Lyme attest to the possibility that I may feel even stronger and more resilient in the days to come, but they also illustrate the possibility that going off antibiotic treatment for more than a few months may mean plunging back into the depths. Time will tell.

25. 63 Days

This painting was an experiment to chart illness and health visually by choosing one dominant image to sum up each day. I wanted to describe "the nature of the beast" to my family so they could be aware of the "two steps forward, one step back" journey of healing. (The bacteria can exist in several forms or stages, such as cysts, and can hide deep inside tissues. Switching to a new medication to smoke them out of hiding or attack them at a different part of their life cycle can cause a sudden die-off called a "Herxheimer" effect – for several days one may plunge back into intense symptoms. It helps to know that this is really a "sign of success." It is also at this point that a person with only a clinical diagnosis of chronic Lyme may at last get a "positive" blood test.) The goal of informing others became secondary to what I received. In creating this calendar I gained the perspective that, even if there were difficult days there would also be easier times ahead, and in spite of pain "life would go on" through Thanksgiving, Christmas, and New Year's Day. This visual reminder helps me have more patience and perspective.

26. Healing Supports

There is no universal protocol for effectively treating Lyme disease. I've heard of people treating it homeopathically, with herbal medicines, ozone steam saunas, hyperbaric oxygen therapy, Rife/Bare machines, and other methods. Everyone I've talked to who is treating it with allopathic medicines is taking different antibiotics on a different schedule, even if they have the same doctor. We're all taking a different batch of supplements and making a variety of differing dietary choices. Some people try many things and don't get well. Others take one prescription for a short time and seem to be cured. It is interesting to hear about other people's successes through different choices, and what they believe in and why. A positive side effect of the epidemic is that more people than ever are having to consider more aspects of the healing process and more of a range of choices to support that healing. It is making people become more self-aware instead of just following a standard prescription and taking "doctor's orders."

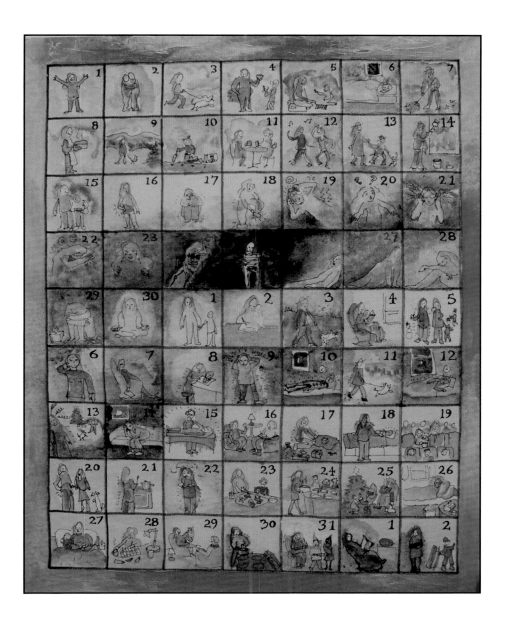

25. 63 Days
acrylic and pen on art board
16" x 20", 2009-2010

I believe everyone who gets Lyme will have their own unique treatment and process of healing, and that this is not likely to change. Lyme, like syphilis, can have many different effects in different parts of the body. There is the compounding issue of co-infections, which may or may not respond to the same treatment as the *Bb* bacteria. Different people's immune systems are in different states of health at the time of initial infection. Furthermore, there is the issue of how long a person may have been ill or misdiagnosed, perhaps allowing time for the invaders to become more deeply entrenched or resistant to certain treatments.

Just "killing germs" isn't enough to make a person well. It's a much more complex process. Professionals such as Dr. Pat Gerbarg and Dr. Richard P. Brown are investigating and sharing the importance of repairing the body's damaged tissues and strengthening the immune system with complimentary herbal medicines, nutritional supplements, and yoga. I have felt it to be very important to address personal, psychological, and spiritual needs to further establish an environment of healing inside and around me. It is beyond the scope of this project for me to explain much more, but there are new books and articles available each year as the epidemic grows, gains attention, and more research is done.

As I contemplate what my body and immune system have been through, I've imagined a different label than "Lyme disease" to describe the situation: "Immune S.O.S." standing for "Immune System Overload Syndrome," in which multiple pathogens and the overall human being is viewed as an out-of-balance microcosm in need of support on many levels, possibly for an extended period of time, possibly with antibiotics, antivirals, and other medications and therapies.

During one of my checkups an intern joined the meeting. As I answered questions my doctor put them in context for him. "That's a typical complaint for Lyme," my doctor would say, "we hear this frequently." I turned to the intern and asked, "So, are you going to become a Lyme Aware doctor, too?" "Nooooo!" He said, raising his hands in a startle reflex, as if "going there" amounted to touching hot coals. At this time most doctors are wary of litigation should they treat their patients with antibiotics

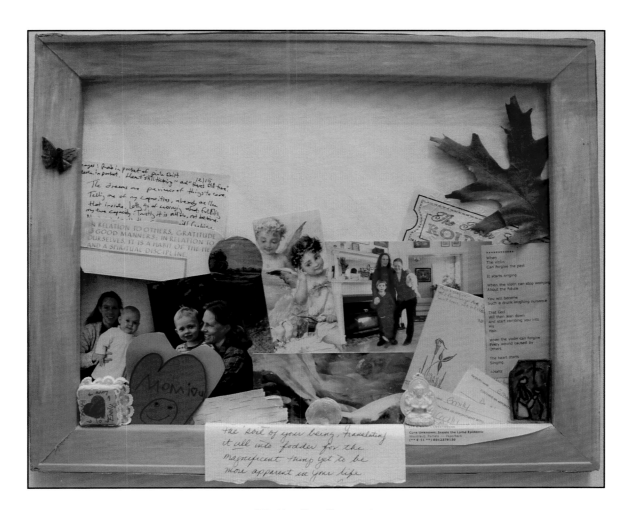

26. Healing Supports
acrylic, photos, paper, wood, lace, glass, leaf, shell, plastic, and bark on canvas and wood
16" x 20", 2010

beyond the official Center for Disease Control's limited protocol. Lyme disease is a highly controversial subject. The documentary *Under Our Skin* examines some of this, as does the book *Cure Unknown*.

I am grateful and full of trust that my doctor is offering me the best information and recommendations available at this time. (Some are acceptable to the insurance company, others are not covered.) I also accept that many choices are left up to me, such as which supplements (and which brands) to take. I believe taking probiotics every night before bed is a must for anyone taking antibiotics for any length of time. My digestion has never been better! I understand that I'm entering the arena at a pioneering level – that everything we're trying is still experimental. My way, so far, has been to research possibilities, discuss choices, and try things that are easily available. I also use intuition to guide me and believe that is part of "taking responsibility" for myself.

Most recently that guidance and intuition led me to the book *Healing Lyme: Natural Healing and Prevention of Lyme*

Borreliosis and Its Coinfections, by Stephen Harrod Buhner (2005). On a day when I was feeling rather low, contemplating some persistent symptoms such as chronic fatigue, I began reading about herbal protocols for treating these symptoms. I felt as if the book were really speaking to me – my fears began to dissolve and I felt a real sense of hope that there are things I can try that I have not already tried. Previously, I had not felt the urge to investigate herbal treatments. Now the time feels right, so that will be my next research project.

One of the biggest changes I've gone through in the learning process with Lyme is that I no longer draw a hard line between the physical and the ephemeral, the world of allopathic medicine and various holistic sects. At this time I'm open to using whatever seems to help and what I feel drawn to trying. Along with a multitude of supplements and prescription medications I have deeply appreciated whatever hands-on support I've been able to afford, such as Therapeutic Massage, Shiatsu, Reiki, CranioSacral Therapy, Osteopathy, and Acupuncture. Here are other things that have been helpful: daily hot baths, with Epsom Salts and Hydrogen Peroxide once or twice a week; hot packs for sore muscles and along the spine; lying down more; short walks; daily sunlight; talking with friends; being cozy with my children; personal reflection and writing time; spiritual study and meditation; counseling to help reprogram my outlook on life and get me out of the post-traumatic-stress-disorder rut; Bach Rescue Remedy; avoiding toxins (especially petrochemicals) by traveling and driving as little as possible and staying out of smelly stores; eating more raw greens, nuts, and seeds, and eating less sugar, dairy, and wheat; eating organic food as much as affordable (not sweating it if I go off some "ideal" diet); and getting subscriptions to Netflix and *The Funny Times* for comic relief!

27. Mindsets

In this exhibit, this is the only piece of art from another era of my life. For me it appears to be a sort of preview or map of many things that have happened since then. I made this collage before I had children and pets, but pictured are images which could represent the core members of my household: a girl, a boy, a dog, and a cat, linked to me by golden threads. I

will not interpret any more, for this was a purely fanciful art-therapy play time that I had alone one day. I see new meaning every time I look at it. That's kind of what the piece is about – looking at things differently, and that the way we look at things can reveal new meaning. The reason this collage made its way into the Lyme-Light exhibit is the idea of mindsets. Having a disease with a neurological component has brought me to the depths of considering mindsets. It has induced me to investigate my thinking and my beliefs about who I am, what I have control over, and what surrender means.

To add further paradox to the discussion of "It's All In Your Head," I believe, after all this expression of gratitude for the help of modern medicine, that healing always begins on the level of the mind. I believe my process of healing began before medication, with the choice to risk reconnecting with life again – my own and others' – and with surrendering to the urgent volition to seek new information and persist in asking for help. This trek through new behavioral territory still takes courage sometimes, but the healing process seems to have a momentum of its own. The more I share, the better life feels.

Instead of trying to hide what I am going through and judging it as "good" or "bad," I'm learning to simply be honest with myself and other people. Coming out of denial is like finally breathing after holding my breath for a long time – breathing into all those old stuck places – breathing into the darkness and breathing back into life.

There are many things we cannot directly control when we are ill, but there are some questions we may ask and some choices we may make about how to look at our lives: What role is this illness playing in my life? What might I learn from it? Who might I be without it? Do I really want to heal? If I begin healing, am I really willing for my life to change in ways I can't predict? Am I open to trying something new, to receiving support from a different source?

Healing may involve different things for different people. It may include stopping playing doctor to oneself at home, finally letting a professional help. It may involve becoming willing to try a new form of treatment outside one's familiar realm of faith and experience. It may entail surrendering into acceptance of illness and pain. It may even include facing the inevitability of death. As one's physical body declines, one may go through a process of coming to peace with one's life and becoming able to experience serenity and spiritual well-being in spite of illness. Healing physically may involve a process of personal empowerment, enduring an initiation process, going on a "hero's journey" that transforms not only one's own life but the very terrain for those who follow.

At this time I have no regrets about the way illness has swerved me away from some experiences and toward others. While illness prevented me from taking certain paths of action, the limitations it imposed skewed me toward the openings I did take, and in those I often flourished. While teaching, for example, my own cognitive struggles have made me sympathetic and sensitive to the unique learning styles of each of my students. Being orally compromised (forgetting words, speaking haltingly) – not all the time, but enough to undermine my confidence to enter certain professional and social arenas – enhanced my focus on visual and written communication.

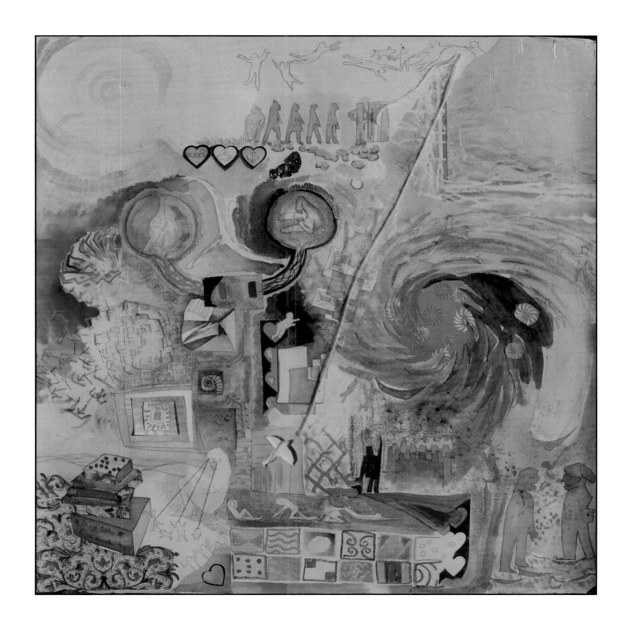

27. Mindsets
watercolor, pencil, crayon,
thread, yarn, staples, and
paper on watercolor paper
22" x 22", 1994

Rather than pressing outward into the world – climbing a career ladder, seeking further formal education, getting into a busy and complicated social life – the conditions of my health have skewed me toward more private, self paced creativity and self-directed study. Through acknowledging (gradually, with setbacks as reminders) my body's need for a low key life style (very little travel or group activities or socializing), I've had more time for quiet reflection and contemplation than most people can carve out in their middle years. My depth of focus on the inner or spiritual life may not have become so intense had I been more able to participate comfortably and successfully in activities out in the world. Nevertheless, besides the effects of chronic illness, I can also look back with gratitude for the amazing journeys I've taken – around the world and within relationships – so, overall I feel I've lived a very rich life.

28. Letting Go

This last painting in the series is about much more than Lyme. In fact, it is symbolic of life beyond Lyme. Letting go of labeling myself as a "Lyme patient" or an "ill person." Letting go of my stories as defining permanent meaning. Letting go of worrying about what effects this story may have in the world. Letting go of the burden of attachment to a particular outcome in return for the freedom of not knowing. Letting go of the need to judge each step of what happens as "failure" or "success." Even letting go of defining this as "a time of healing."

This image also illustrates a wonderful paradox that one may experience on many levels: that sometimes when something is let go of, it ceases to have substance any longer. Even something as consuming as pain, as heavy as guilt, as dwarfing as shame, as monstrous as fear, as solid as ignorance, can dissolve into thin air and become nothing. If transformation is truly desired, much is possible beyond the limits of our rational understanding. In spite of and even through illness, there can be opening of hearts and minds.

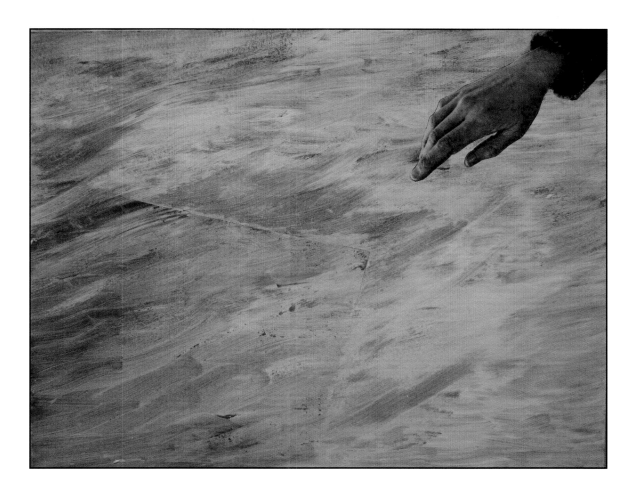

28. Letting Go
acrylic and paper on art board
16" x 20", 2010

Acknowledgements

First, I offer my warmest gratitude to my family, friends, and community for your emotional, financial, and artistic support – this project has been a joint venture, with several people playing more than one important role. This is by no means an exhaustive list. In particular, thank you Mary and Paul Gloger – a.k.a. "Mama and Papa" – for helping fund the first printing and joining me in the difficult yet amazing process of revisiting and revaluing the past. Thank you Papa for your impeccable editing support. Thank you Hana Bracale, Andreas Doerfler, and Mama for your invaluable design, editing, layout, and marketing advice. In the beginning, thank you career counselors Glenon Friedmann and Jill Barlow-Kelly for telling me to "rest first" – the paintings soon followed. Thanks artist, teacher, and Lyme survivor Ernie McMullen for your advice to seek medical help and to explore painting even with brain fog. Thank you reporters Jessica Bloch, Bob Evans, Donna Gold, Robert Levin, and Nan Lincoln for your sensitive coverage of the original Lyme-Light exhibit. Thank you Susan Lerner, Terry Watson, Arthur and Carol Westing, Ed Synder, and everyone who signed the exhibit guest log, for assuring me this work was of value and should be widely shared. Thank you Aaron Steiner and then Andreas Doerfler for designing, hosting, and managing the Lyme-Light website. Thank you Jane Karker, president of Maine Authors Publishing for your professional enthusiasm and personal conviction that this work should also be shared as a book, and to art director David Allen. Kind regards to the woman at AMC who stayed at the table and listened, helping me find my soul's bearings to begin this book project. Thank you doctor, teacher, author and Lyme survivor Pat Gerbarg for writing the foreword to usher it in. My creative work also rests on a foundation of support from my community on Mount Desert Island, my neighbors on Glen Mary Road, and friends and family far and near who have helped me find perspective, comfort, courage, and humor during sickness and in health – especially Aubrey Bart, John Henry Bart, Regina Bernhardt, Ann Bohrer, Dennis Bracale, Hana Bracale, Danette Burchill, Andreas Doerfler, Georgia Douillet, Dawn Dreisbach, Sue Haynes, Betsey Holtzmann, Yvonne Maiden, Margarita Marnik, Heather Nuesslein, Pam Roland, Aaron Steiner, and Phyllis Weliver. Hugs to my "Lyme Sisters" Linda Adams, Meg Burden, Malia and Rose Demers, Nina Devenney, Happy Dickey, Beth Lambert, Kirsten Stockman, and Daaby Tingle. Thanks to Lisa Burton and Chris Vincenty of Reel Pizza for hosting the movie fundraiser, and cheers to everyone who came. My well-being has also been supported by the care of healers and counselors who have helped me find comfort and alignment on many levels. Thank you Kathleeen Bowman, Michael Curless, Steve Curtin, Anna Durand, Diane Fehrenbach, Matt Gerrish, Jessie Greenbaum, Linette Grindal, Julie Havener, Sandy Bart Heimann, Cecily Judd, Kathleen Kotas, Deborah Loftus, Sheridy Olson, Deborah Page, Dan Torinus, Charly Weir, and Susan Whittaker. I am most grateful to my doctor and fellow clarinetist Meryl Nass, whose professional care and personal encouragement helped restore my ability and willingness to be here.

About the Author and Artist

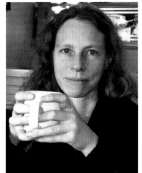

Emily Bracale is an artist, writer, teacher, and Reiki Master Teacher, with a B.A. in Human Ecology from College of the Atlantic. She grew up in Michigan and attended the Interlochen Arts Academy. She now lives in Bar Harbor, Maine. To see her art online go to the Art/Maine Artists Guild link at www.davistownmuseum.org, and www.inthelyme-light.com.

Photo by Hana Bracale